ACUPUNCTURE

Is it for you?

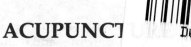

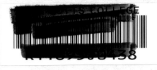

Professor J R Worsley has over thirty years experience
in the field of acupuncture and is the founder
of the College of Traditional Chinese Acupuncture (UK)
and the Traditional Acupuncture Institute (USA).

ACUPUNCTURE

Is it for you?

J R Worsley

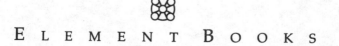

ELEMENT BOOKS

© J R Worsley 1988

First Published in 1973

First UK edition published in 1985
This revised edition first published in 1988 by
Element Books Limited
Longmead, Shaftesbury, Dorset

Second impression 1990

Text designed by Humphrey Stone
Cover design by Max Fairbrother
Cover Illustration: Burt Glinn - Magnum Photos
Printed and bound in Great Britain by
Billings Ltd, Hylton Road, Worcester

British Library Cataloguing in Publication Data
Worsley, J.R.
Acupuncture: Is it for you?
1. Acupuncture
I. Title
615.8'92

ISBN 1-85230-047-7

Contents

5   The Use of Needles   36

6   The Use of Moxa and Other Treatments   41

7   Types of Illness Helped by Acupuncture   44

Appendix Two: Acupuncture in the United States of America

Preface

It is my earnest belief that traditional Chinese acupuncture is one of the most wonderful systems of healing. It is one which has truly stood the test of time. Like all other systems it has certain limitations but these are indeed few. It must nevertheless be emphasized that acupuncture is not a panacea, a cure for everything; furthermore, the results achieved will depend to a great extent upon the quality of training, the skill and the experience of the practitioner.

I also believe that all the available systems of medical treatment – be it Western medicine, homoeopathy, osteopathy, naturopathy, herbalism, acupuncture or whatever – have an important part to play in healing the sick. No one system, when practised in its true tradition, is any better or worse than another.

Whilst it must be said that a system of medicine is only as good as the person who practises it, it is also important to say that neither man nor woman can cure any disease. Only Nature can cure disease. Practitioners only assist Nature, acting as instruments of Nature in putting the patient back on the path to health.

Since the first edition of this book, published twelve years ago, I am pleased to be able to say that many people have told me that they found it both interesting and informative, and that they were delighted with the clear way in which the contents were laid out. However, there were also suggestions that I might helpfully modify and extend the book to provide a little more insight into the concepts which lie at the foundation of this system. Thus, in this edition, I have decided to retain that part of the former edition which deals with the questions most frequently asked about acupuncture and have used again the simple question and answer format. But I have also included, as requested, some of the ideas, concepts and laws which underlie diagnosis and treatment in Chinese traditional medicine.

I do wish it to be borne in mind, however, that I do not in any way intend this book to be regarded as a text of guidance – either for someone seeking to practise this medicine on others, or for anyone seeking to diagnose the symptoms of disease (either his or her own, or those of others). I cannot stress strongly enough that this system of medicine is very powerful and needs to be studied in depth very carefully, under skilled guidance, in order that it may be practised safely. What I have tried to do is share with you some of the wisdom and joy of traditional Chinese medicine. In doing so, I hope that you will be able to learn something – be it only a little – about the nature of your own body, mind and spirit.

I also wish to emphasize that this knowledge is not something that I have discovered. I am simply telling you about the art and science of a system of healing which has not changed in the last five thousand years – and which will not change in the next five thousand years because it is based entirely on natural laws which will never change. Neither man nor woman can improve on Nature.

I also hope that the book will increase the reader's awareness of how Man interacts with Nature, and how this awareness is important for the maintenance of health. The latter part of the book contains much about the way we in the West tend to live our lives and how, as a result, body, mind and spirit can become sick. I think we should be aware of these reasons. If we are to maintain our good health, it is most important that we, individually, should adjust our ways of living as far as possible in order to eliminate or lessen the stresses to which we become subject in the modern world. Acupuncture can do much to help fight and prevent disease; but maintaining health is not solely the responsibility of the doctor or practitioner; for the most part it is our own.

Finally, I would like to express my gratitude to Julia Measures for her valuable assistance in the compiling of this book; also for the help given in its preparation by my son, John, and by John Moore.

J R WORSLEY

Royal Leamington Spa, 1985

Foreword

I am grateful to have the opportunity to write the foreword to this book so that I can share my personal experience of traditional Chinese acupuncture under the guidance of J.R. – my teacher, friend and healer.

As a practising plastic surgeon in the United States, I began my study of acupuncture with Professor Worsley in 1972 at the College of Traditional Chinese Acupuncture in England. It was my original intention to learn how to perform acupuncture anaesthesia as an adjunct to my surgical practice but I soon became aware that traditional acupuncture provided a way of viewing life and the human body which was totally different from the one I had received in medical school some twenty-one years before.

For three years I practised both acupuncture and surgery. I then became so involved with the former that I gave up the latter and planned to go around the world to look at alternative forms of healing before undertaking further acupuncture study. Shortly after leaving my surgical practice, I was involved in a catastrophic automobile accident in California in which I suffered fractures of my right arm, left leg, pelvis, ribs and skull. My healing was delayed by many complications. Although I could walk and talk, I was left with moderate brain damage. I was unable to function well enough to resume productive work. My defects included a moderately severe, short-term memory loss, some loss of inductive reasoning and difficulty with balance. The doctors who treated me told me I would have to live with these defects as nothing more could be done.

After two years, my condition had not significantly changed

and I decided to return to England to be treated by Professor Worsley with traditional acupuncture. Within six weeks most of my symptoms had cleared but it required another six months of treatment to make the improvement permanent.

As one who had been trained as an allopathic physician, I had been fascinated to observe and evaluate the emotional, mental and physical changes my patients underwent when I treated them with traditional acupuncture; but for me to experience these changes as the patient was almost indescribable. To me it was a miracle to be brought back to a functioning level in that very brief period of time – by means of just a single physical technique of inserting thin, sharp, almost painless needles through the skin.

The concepts of traditional Chinese acupuncture are foreign to Western thought. As a master of this form of healing, Professor Worsley has in this book presented, in a clear, concise way, the basic principles of traditional acupuncture. The concept that our good health depends on the balance of the Life-Force energy (*Ch'i*) in our bodies is discussed in a way that is easy to understand. It is most beneficial to have knowledge of this ancient system of healing for it provides an alternative approach to the promotion of health and to the treatment of those disease processes which do not respond well to Western medicine.

Through his teaching, and through his book, Professor Worsley has opened this path to many, and I am pleased to be one of those whose life has been enriched by contact with him.

MARCY GOLDSTEIN, M.D.
St. Louis, Missouri, U.S.A.

1   What is Acupuncture?

Acupuncture is one of the oldest forms of healing known to mankind. It originated in China nearly five thousand years ago. The fact that it is still being practised today speaks much for the efficacy of this treatment and for the truth of the principles on which it is based. These principles relate to the Order of Nature (the way the universe works). The observation and knowledge of the principles can be seen to underlie the whole of Chinese culture, including all traditional Chinese medical thinking.

The application of these principles to the health of the human body was first written down – about 200 BC or a little earlier, during a golden age of Chinese thought – in a book that remains the foundation of all Chinese medicine (of which acupuncture and moxabustion are an important part). This book, the *Nei Ching* – the Yellow Emperor's Classic of Internal Medicine – is a treatise on life itself. As well as explaining how to live one's life in accordance with the great natural laws of the universe, and examining at length the normal functions of the human body, and bodily diseases and their causes, the *Nei Ching* sets out for the first time the theory on which the whole of acupuncture is based. This is the 'meridian theory' which concerns the flow of life-energy through the body. (This will be discussed in the next chapter).

Acupuncture and moxabustion treatment assists nature by influencing this energy in such a way that it may return to its natural flow and balance in a person. This allows body, mind and spirit to return to health. The influence is achieved by inserting very fine needles into specific points on the body, or by burning a herb *(artemisia vulgaris latiflora)* on these points. This burning of the herb is referred to as moxabustion.

When I speak of acupuncture I am referring to traditional Chinese acupuncture, or Chinese classical acupuncture to give it its more accurate name. It is a complex system of healing and takes a considerable number of years to learn; and very many more to gain expertise and wisdom.

A practitioner of traditional Chinese acupuncture has certain aims in mind when treating a patient. These are:

To treat the patient as a whole. This means that the practitioner considers the physical body, the mind and the spirit together as a whole; as a unity. He or she considers this unity as a part of the whole creation, having its own very individual and unique relationship with its environment.

To seek the cause of the disease. It is most important that the manifest complaint itself should not be considered the prime concern. The complaint is really only a distress signal (or symptom) of the disease. The acupuncturist will try to find the underlying reason why the disease is present. He or she will therefore need to understand the nature of the energy imbalance that has occurred, and to find out whereabouts and in what way the natural flow and balance of energy has broken down. The cause of the breakdown can be physical, mental or spiritual.

Having found the seat of the energy imbalance, to correct the cause of the problem. When the energy is restored to balance and harmony, and is flowing throughout the body as nature ordained, the symptoms of the illness will start to disappear (without there necessarily having been special treatment of the symptoms themselves). To help the patient deal with the cause of the disease, it is important that he or she should understand, if possible, the underlying reason for the illness. There can then be the possibility of altering situations which may, by their very nature, have generated the disease.

To help the patient get well and stay well. The patient has to take some responsibility in this process. (This will be

2

discussed later in the chapter on disease and its prevention).

A practitioner of traditional acupuncture must strive to see patients not just as they are at the time of examination but as they would be if they were whole and perfect in body, mind and spirit, with every possibility of their 'unique being' realized. The personality and behaviour of a person when ill will not necessarily be true to his or her own real nature; it may indeed be very different. The work of the doctor of traditional Chinese acupuncture is to help the sick person to become renewed, revitalized and brought to the fullness of their potential.

It should be pointed out that not all acupuncturists practise the traditional Chinese acupuncture referred to here. Many use acupuncture to treat the symptom rather than concern themselves with the cause. I feel it is important for a prospective patient to understand the difference between these two methods and to be aware of the dangers of symptomatic acupuncture. (This is discussed in chapter 10).

Finally, acupuncture can also be used for analgesia to replace conventional anaesthetics during an operation or for dentistry. (This, too, is discussed at some length in chapter 10).

2   How Acupuncture Works

Why does acupuncture work? What happens when you bring about this balance in a person's energy that you mentioned earlier?

Traditional Chinese medicine states that it is the vital force, the life force, in the body that controls the workings of the main organs and systems of the body. This vital force, or *Ch'i* energy as the Chinese call it, circulates from one organ to another along channels or pathways termed meridians, always following a certain route.

There are twelve of these meridians, each of them feeding one of the main organs or functions of the body – heart, small intestine, bladder, kidney, circulation-sex, three heater, gall bladder, liver, lungs, colon, stomach and spleen. In order that each and all of these organs may be healthy, and working properly and in harmony with each other, the *Ch'i* energy must be flowing freely and in the correct strength and quality through each of the meridians. It is, in fact, impossible to be ill in body, mind or spirit if the energy within the twelve meridians is balanced and harmonious. In all illness the energy is out of balance. The pain, or symptom, is a distress signal notifying us of this imbalance, be it due to a physical, mental or spiritual cause.

Thus acupuncture treatment sets out to correct any imbalance in the energy of a person. The aim is to restore the energy to its natural balance and flow and to re-establish its rhythm with the natural cycles of day and night, the seasons, the time of day. Harmony and equilibrium are then re-established within the body, within the mind, within the spirit of the person, and between the person and the environment. As the energy imbalances are corrected, the person's body, mind and spirit start to heal.

This explains very briefly what is happening when acupuncture is used. In order to bring about health we balance the energy.

How can the acupuncturist bring about this balance by the use of needles and moxa?

Acupuncture directly controls the energy at special points located on the meridians (the energy pathways). When gently inserted into these acupuncture points, the needles produce various effects. According to the manipulation of the needles, the energy is either drawn to a meridian, or dispersed from it.

This change in energy, as a result of the acupuncture treatment, is confirmed in many ways. Initially, from a pulse change; and then there will also be colour changes, emotional changes, etcetera, which I will explain in more detail later. The purpose of mentioning the changes here is to illustrate that they are clearly evident and can be observed and measured. On many occasions patients themselves are aware of a change in their well being: for example, pain may diminish, which again indicates that the balance of the *Ch'i* energy is coming nearer to normal.

Why did the energy get out of balance in the first place?

This question really could be construed as 'Why do people become sick in the first place?' I will be describing the reasons for the cause of disease and sickness later.

One of the great joys of traditional Chinese acupuncture is that, irrespective of the disease or symptom, once we are able to find the cause of the energy imbalance and correct it, then those symptoms and the sickness will disappear.

Can the person be restored to health if the factor causing the disease is still there?

Yes and no. The treatment in itself often appears to be enough. If the organs and the functions can get strong again and return to normal, and the patient is feeling so much better, then frequently they find themselves better able to deal with situations which, during their sickness, would have over-whelmed them. They are often able to see things more clearly when they are healthier; and thus they are able to make better and wiser decisions in relation to their life style. For example, some may change their occupations. Some may express grief that they have been hiding or pushing aside. Some will be able to come to terms in relationships. All things that before treat-ment they had not been strong enough in themselves to deal with.

However, there are occasions when we need to direct and encourage a patient to make necessary changes – be these in diet, life style, exercise – before the treatments can hold and before long-term healing can take place. It was, and still is, an important part of the role of the practitioner of traditional acupuncture to help to guide the patient towards the *Tao* (the Chinese way of Wholeness, see chapter 13), the basis of a healthy life.

3 How the Energy Imbalance in a Person is Assessed: *Yin-Yang and the Five Elements*

What is meant by the energy being in harmony and balance? How can the practitioner measure this?

The Chinese have developed a system by which they can read the state of a person's energy. This system is based on *yin* and *yang* and the five elements – principles that underlie the whole of Chinese culture. They have arisen from direct observation. The ancient Chinese were keenly aware of Nature and watched her closely. They observed that things were always changing, and that we on this earth are inevitably affected also by certain cycles of change. The most obvious of these are day and night and the cycle of seasons throughout a year.

YIN-YANG

The Chinese saw that the energy of creation was always moving between two extremes – as with day and night, summer and winter, life and death. It is like energy moving between the two poles of a battery, between the positive and the negative. One pole cannot exist without the other. The Chinese called these polarities of *Ch'i* energy *yin* and *yang*. They came to see them at work in everything.

To give a flavour of what these terms mean without getting too technical, *yang* can in its simplest form be represented by sun, warmth, expansion, day, heat and male, whereas *yin* can be represented by night, cold, stillness and female. If we look a little further we can see the interplay of *yin* and *yang* at a slightly deeper level. For example, when the sun is shining, then *yang* would be represented by the sunny side of the mountain and *yin* would be represented by the shady side of the mountain. This would be a predominantly *yang* situation – daytime, light, sun; but the *yin* is present too – in the shades, the clouds. The same can be said of the night, which, in our earlier classification we called *yin*. The light from the stars becomes the *yang* within the *yin*. The full moon itself casts light upon the earth thus creating a brighter, light side and a dark side of the mountain. Here we have both the *yin* and the *yang* expressed in a predominantly *yin* situation.

It is important to understand the balance and harmony between *yin* and *yang*. Both are necessary. One is not better than the other. They are both always there, always flowing and moving and balancing each other. We see day flow into night, sunshine flow into shadow, and so on. This intermingling and changing of *yin* and *yang* is everywhere and in everything.

The Chinese saw the importance of this balance, not only within nature but also within the human being. They looked to see if there was a harmonious mingling and flowing of these two qualities of energy in a person, both the sunshine and the shade. Was a person able to be active, energetic, warm, friendly, outgoing? Was he or she able to be passive, receptive, to rest, to go inward to be refreshed?

The Chinese observed that if either *yin* or *yang* becomes over-dominant, then the person becomes unhealthy. The person who is always working and never rests will finally collapse. The person who gets more and more depressed and inward-looking, and loses all ability to turn outwards again, will become physically ill.

So here we have our first main key for knowing whether a person's energy is out of balance. We look to see whether there is an excess or a deficiency of either the *yin* or the *yang* qualities in a person.

THE FIVE ELEMENTS

The Chinese then took their observations a step further. They noted the cycle of five seasons – spring, summer, late summer, autumn and winter. And they saw how those seasons expressed different stages of the movement from *yin* to *yang* and from *yang* to *yin*. For example, in the spring and summer the energy is rising and is active, and is predominantly *yang*. And in the autumn and the winter the energy is withdrawing, becoming passive and inward, and becomes predominantly *yin*. Each of the seasons of the year has its own particular quality, has its own flavour and its own unique being. And the Chinese observed that there were five of these major changes of quality and function of the energy throughout the year – hence the five seasons.

For example, we can readily see that the season of spring is one of birth and growth. This can be seen as the seeds begin to come alive and the plants start to burst upward, and to grow. There is a feeling of re-birth and excitement in the air.

In summer, the sun is warming the earth and caressing the plants, encouraging them towards their fullness and their maturity.

The later summer is the season when the intensity of the summer sun is accompanied by a gentle, welcoming breeze. This is the season of harvest, where there is the reaping of what has been sown, in accordance with the natural laws of nature.

The autumn is a season when the leaves begin to fall to the earth from whence they came. The trees that were heavily-laden with leaves and fruit are now ready to discard all their finery and to bare themselves in preparation for the following year.

The winter is a season of withdrawal. The activity of all the previous four seasons is now slowed down. Throughout these seasons we see different activities; but then, in the winter, there is a resting period.

The Chinese saw in this cycle of the seasons the manifestation of the great principle of creation. They saw the great flowing of energy, of creation, as it moves from *yin* to *yang*, and back to *yin*. From stillness to activity, and back to stillness; from death to life, and from life to death; and it is all done in an orderly way as it moves through the five stages that we see in the seasons. Each stage has its own particular quality which we can recognise – five great steps of the creative energy, the five elements. The Chinese called the five elements Wood, Fire, Earth, Metal and Water.

9

Don't be worried by these names. They are merely labels used to describe the different qualities of the vital *Ch'i* energy that flows within every one of us. The laws that I have just explained as working outside in nature are the same laws that are controlling the energy within ourselves. It is perhaps confusing at first to find that names of things that are tangible should have been used to describe that which is intangible. But these were the terms that were used by the Chinese, and they are still used today because, as we shall see, they convey the appropriate qualities which we can appreciate.

Thus, in the springtime, the energy of the creative cycle is in the phase that the Chinese call Wood. We can know the quality of this Wood energy by considering the season of spring. This energy expresses itself in birth and growth, and in the hope for future harvest. We can see this in the season of spring outside, but we can also see this same element of energy within each and every one of us. We can see it in a person's own birth and growth, in his or her hopes for the future, in the ability to give birth to ideas and projects, and so on.

In the summer, the creative activity of the energy expresses itself in a special way that the Chinese called Fire. The Fire energy expresses itself in the warmth of the summer sun, and we can see this element too within the human being because the Fire energy is concerned with the warmth within a person – joy, love and compassion.

The quality of the Earth element is that of the mother – mother earth, the caring, loving provider. The same provider as the human mother providing for her child, with food and love and warmth for the mind, body and spirit.

The element Metal is like the autumn. As the trees let go of the leaves when the work is done for the year, so there is a need within to discard what has been finished with and to let go of labours until the next spring time, or the next new beginning. It is the element which is responsible within for the removal of poisons and toxins, and the waste matter that needs to be discarded. It is also the element concerned with quality itself. As the Earth element is the mother, the Metal element is the father. As the world becomes bared of its greenness in the autumn, there is a return to the inner spirit, to the heavens, to the father. In the autumn of a person's life, he or she often turns to matters of the spirit and sets out on a new path – an inner path, a path more meaningful to that individual.

The quality of the element Water can be seen in winter. It is the element responsible for the collection and the storage of fluids. As the rains fall down the mountain-sides and are channelled into rivers and reservoirs – to provide us with water throughout the following year and through the intensity of the heat of the summer – so does the element Water within provide our bodies with all of its necessary fluids and secretions.

So this cycle of the elements that we see in the seasons can also be seen within us. We can all grow, warm others, be warmed by others; and be provided for, and be guided. And when the period of rest comes, we can look back and count our blessings and can look forward to the challenge of another year. We can know by the natural progression of the seasons that, if we are obedient to the laws of Nature in relation to the seasons, then each year as we plough and sow, so there will be a harvest, ultimate joy, and connection with both our mother and our father.

But let us look at what happens if the seasons, or the elements, become imbalanced. If, for example, during the summer there were no warmth at all, no sun and no heat, then the crops would not ripen and the harvest would be doomed to fail. The earth would be cold and thus would not be able to provide the fruits. In ancient times this would have meant starvation for those depending upon the crop for their food during the ensuing months.

If we now take that deprivation as an analogy for the element Fire within, we can see that if there is no heat, no fire within a human being, then without love, without compassion and understanding, without warmth within himself, he will not be able to reap a harvest. Thus, as in the outer world, the earth within him would become barren and cold, and his life as a result would be as empty as the physical granaries.

This cycle of the five elements is the second major principle by which the Chinese assess the state of a person's energy. They read whether all five elements are working together in balance and harmony, or whether any one of them has become out of balance with the others. Is there too much or too little of the quality of Fire – and so on?

I have now described the principles of *yin* and *yang* and the five elements, and how the Chinese observed them at work in everything. They did not see any difference between the energy outside man and the energy inside man. It is the one life force moving through the whole of creation, and moving through all life on this earth. Any alteration in the *Ch'i* energy observable in our environment will also be seen in the *Ch'i* energy of our bodies. Most people can feel the rising energy of the springtime within themselves for example. We are in tune with *yin* and *yang* and with the cycle of energy of the five elements manifesting in the seasons. This means that we are able to look at these cycles of *yin* and *yang* and the five elements within a person, and can see when they become out of balance.

Can you say something more of how you would see the five elements manifesting in a man or a woman?

Each of the five elements is expressing itself in everything. There are certain aspects of us that are particularly useful in giving very direct information about the state of the elements. These are the emotions, sound of voice, colour of face, and odour of the body. We can get additional information, for example, from stated preferences for certain flavours of food, the like or dislike of certain colours and particular times of the day. Each of the elements has direct correspondence not only in the physical body but, perhaps more importantly, in the mental and spiritual aspects of ourselves also.

To illustrate these points, I ask you to remember the meridians or energy pathways which I mentioned earlier. Two of the twelve meridians are under the dominion of the Wood energy. The energy in a particular meridian controls the working of a certain organ and function; in this case, the two Wood organs are the liver and the gall bladder. Wood also controls the functions of the eyes and our vision, and controls the state of the nails, ligaments and tendons.

Emotionally, Wood controls anger.

If we recall the description of the quality of spring, I spoke about new growth and of hope for the future. The two Wood meridians affect our ability to deal with these aspects of our lives – to provide enterprise and hope for the future.

Someone brought up in the Western world may have difficulty at first in understanding the qualities of the elements. The ancient Chinese had a very beautiful way of explaining how they manifest in us on all levels of our being. They compared the controlling function of an element to a Minister of State. Each meridian was said to be under the control of a special 'Minister' who had particular functions within the unified body, mind and spirit.

Thus the Ministers for the two Wood element meridians were the Official of Planning (liver) and the Official of Decision-Making and Judgement (gall bladder). They were in charge of these functions in the whole person at all levels.

This may at first sound a little fantastic but closer scrutiny will show that wisdom was inherent in this idea.

Let us return again to consideration of the springtime, to the quality of the spring and the Wood energy. As I have said, it is a time of new birth, of hope, of planning for the future months. Here we can see the Officials of Planning and Decision-Making at work. It is in the springtime of our lives that we need to make plans for our future, our direction, our work. At the birth of a new idea, a new scheme, we need to plan and make decisions. Our holiday this year, for example, will really begin when we have our first ideas, decide where to go and make plans.

Perhaps now you can see why it makes sense that the Wood energy controls the eyes and the vision. We need our physical eyes to see what is going on, and our 'inner eye' to be able to envisage the future. We need our mental vision to make wise and correct decisions as we move forward into the future.

So, these Wood officials are concerned with seeing in all ways – physically, mentally, spiritually. We hear people say, 'I just don't know what to do; I can't see straight;' or 'I can't see my way to making a decision.'

Or consider what happens if we feel there is no future for us. Don't we feel hopeless, become shut off and withdrawn, blind to possibilities?

So we see how vision is involved in all senses of the word. In this situation are we not likely to feel irritable and easily angry? Isn't it understandable that we soon become angry with a world that seems to offer us no future, no hope? Again, we may well feel angry if we make the wrong plans and decisions, and get ourselves into difficult situations.

So hope and anger are part of the natural expression of the energy of the Wood element.

As I stated before, the two Wood meridians are called the liver meridian and the gall bladder meridian. Each is named after the main organ that it directly feeds and has responsibility for. It is unfortunate, perhaps, that they are named in this physical way, because we in the West are inclined to direct our thoughts only to the organ itself. But as I have explained, the meridian indicates far more than that; it concerns itself with all the subtle aspects of a particular function throughout the whole body, mind and spirit.

I could describe all the elements and their meridians in this way, but I hope that this one example will give you some insight into how the Chinese understand the five elements, and their relationships within the oneness of everything. Man and woman are in tune with that oneness when in a state of health. When we are alienated or taken away from that oneness by elemental unbalance, we are subject to disease.

Thus, in the case of the Wood meridians, if these are not functioning properly as nature ordained, if they are not in balance, then the aspects that I described as being expressions of the Wood energy will become imbalanced and fail in their functioning.

We will expect to find the liver or gall bladder, or both, not functioning properly. Disease may not have developed too far physically, but we may expect there to be trouble with the eyes or the vision – mental vision as well as physical vision. The nails may show signs of ill-health – being hard, brittle, thick, soft, ridged. The ligaments may be in trouble, causing aching, stiffness, constriction. The person may become very angry. Perhaps he may become very confused because he cannot plan or make decisions; and his ability to give birth to the new growth, new ideas, and to have hope for the future may be impaired. In these ways we are able to see that the Wood element is out of balance.

Each element is expressing itself through everything and, by understanding these elements, we gain direct information about the person. We know too that, when imbalance occurs, a specific odour is emitted from the body, and the sound of the voice and the colour of the face expresses it. We can note how the person has been drawn to eat certain foods, sometimes excesses of them; or even how he has turned away from what he has hitherto preferred. We can see how he may enjoy one season and hate others; how he may feel better at one time of day compared with the rest of the day, and how he may feel worse at one time of the day compared with the rest of the day. These things help us in diagnosis and help us later to assess the effect of our treatment. This is something that is very special in traditional Chinese acupuncture.

In Western medicine we have a fine system of diagnosis which improves continually, but there is no instruction built into that diagnosis as to how to treat the underlying problem. In traditional Chinese acupuncture the diagnosis instructs the practitioner as to how to treat the underlying cause – in accordance with the natural laws. So if we diagnose an imbalance in the Wood energy, then the treatment will simply be to restore it to balance – to re-establish its balance with the other elements.

The person will then start to get better and the symptoms will begin to disappear. Not only will the liver and the gall bladder start to function better but the eyes and vision, the nails and ligaments will improve. The person will feel less irritable, and anger will be under better control. The person will feel more hopeful and better able to face the future. He or she will make a better job of planning and of decision-making. Any excess of shouting will leave the voice, and any craving for sour food will diminish. Excessive love or hate of the spring will level out to normal. All these signs of distress will start to disappear as the Wood energy comes into balance and harmony with the other elements.

You asked me how one can see the five elements showing in a man or a woman. I have used the Wood element as an example, showing how it can be seen in someone when it is both in balance and out of balance. Similarly, we can see the other four elements manifesting in a person, properly or otherwise.

I have also shown how the acupuncturist looks at the energy in a person and sees whether it is in balance and harmony in relation to two principles – the *yin* and *yang* and the five elements. This observation of the elemental state in a person forms the basis of the acupuncturist's diagnosis and selection of treatment.

4 The Acupuncture Practitioner's Method of Diagnosis: *How a more Detailed Assessment of a Patient's Energy is Made*

Does the acupuncture practitioner use different methods of diagnosis from those normally used by a Western doctor?

Yes, indeed. As I have already explained when talking about energy balance and imbalance, diagnosis in Chinese medicine means discovering the type of energy imbalance within a particular person. The practitioner needs to discover and evaluate which element first became imbalanced and then to go further to find which meridian within that element was the first to become imbalanced.

Thus he is looking for something very different from an orthodox Western doctor when carrying out his examination. He is not seeking to diagnose the manifest physical disease syndrome but to discover the energetic imbalance that has given rise to that syndrome. The symptom – whether it be high blood pressure, hardening of the arteries, frozen shoulder, migraine, or whatever – is not of particular importance in itself. It is useful information, but not directly relevant to the basic diagnosis. To label known symptoms does not tell you how to treat the cause.

So the traditional Chinese doctor wants to discover the elemental energy imbalance which has given rise to the high blood pressure, the frozen shoulder or migraine. This diagnosis will give him exact information about how to proceed with the treatment.

How can the acupuncture practitioner tell which element was the first to become imbalanced? What does he look for?

I explained earlier how the Wood element will show itself in a person if it is imbalanced. Unfortunately traditional diagnosis is not that simple. It is very rare to find a person exhibiting symptoms simply of one-element imbalance. He or she may well be showing signs of imbalance in perhaps two or three elements because imbalance in one element will most likely upset one or two of the others. Thus, supposing there is evidence that there is a Water imbalance, a Wood imbalance and a Fire imbalance. The art of traditional diagnosis is then to determine which of them is the *primary* imbalance. If the practitioner then works on the primary imbalance, the other two elements will correct themselves.

To discover the primary energy imbalance, the traditional Chinese acupuncturist is trained to use four basic techniques. He is looking for the manifestations of the energy imbalance (such as I spoke about in relation to the Wood element) through four basic means of obtaining information.

ASKING

By this method he will find out the description and history of the problem – the manifest symptoms of the trouble, when and how they started, and what has been done up to that point by way of treatment. He will want a full medical history plus a general picture of the patient's life – for example, any times of recent or past stress, injury, sickness, emotional upset, previous disease, matters relating to experiences in childhood, relationships within the family circle, and so on. This family history is important because the first element to become imbalanced may have started to become so very early in the patient's life, manifesting then through certain illnesses or emotional disturbances. As the years have passed, that will have caused other elements to become strained and imbalanced.

The practitioner will also ask the patient about many other things I have already mentioned. The questions may not seem to have any bearing upon the physical symptom but they are in fact designed to find the primary *cause* of the symptom. There-fore the patient should not be surprised to find that during this examination he is asked, for example, questions as to how he feels about the various seasons of the year, about different times of day, about the weather, and about specific likes and dislikes in the way of food. There will be questions relating to occupation, to parents, to schooling – the list is extensive. What the practitioner is endeavouring to do is to assess the state of the mind and the spirit as well as the physical body because treating the symptom of the physical body only is merely palliation, and may do little or nothing towards restor-ing the patient to full health. This is why the initial examina-tion can take from two to three hours. We cannot be sure of returning the body, mind and spirit to health unless we can be sure of the cause.

HEARING

Hearing is the second way the acupuncturist elicits informa-tion. There are two major things to listen for. The first is the actual sound of the voice, and as I have said previously, if the Wood energy is imbalanced then he will hear a sound of 'shouting' in the patient's voice (or possibly that there is a complete absence of shouting at all times). Thus the patient not only shouts when he gets angry, which of course would be appropriate and healthy, but he also shouts at inappropriate times – perhaps when he is telling about something which he has really enjoyed, or when he is really sad.

The second thing is to listen to the actual words that the person uses and how they are spoken. The practitioner listens to how the person expresses himself or herself. Does he or she speak fluently, haltingly, with a stammer, with uncertainty, with fear, with apprehension? I have already mentioned how word and sound can give a clue to the elemental imbalances. I mentioned that Wood energy controls the eyes and the vision, and how a patient with Wood imbalance may say 'I just can't see what to do', 'I can't see the wood for the trees', 'I don't see any hope for the future.' These very words may well indicate the trouble so that the practitioner may then want to look closely at the element Wood and the two organs associated with this element.

Also he will not only evaluate from the sounds that are heard but from the patient's body-position and the attitude of the patient while he or she is actually talking. The practitioner may hear or see at one level, and yet from listening and looking more subtly, he can see that this evidence is not really truthful at a deeper level. This manifest behaviour is not how the patient really feels inside. For example – as can be observed in everyday life – Miss X may be feeling quite wretched inside and quite unhappy, and yet when she meets an acquaintance walking down the street who asks, 'Hello, young lady, how are you?', she replies, 'Oh, I'm wonderful, thank you.' The average person would probably accept what she has said as being true. A trained practitioner would be able to see and hear that Miss X was presenting a mask. He would know the way she really felt – from the way that she was making the reply, from the way that she said it. He would see she was wishing others to hear one thing but inside she was feeling something quite opposite.

Before going further, it should be said that these examples are not quite as simple as I may seem to be making them out to be. I am endeavouring to give just a basic understanding of the methods used in acupuncture diagnosis. In practice diagnosis is far more complicated. The Wood manifestations I have given can also emanate via any one of the organs, or any one of the elements; this can only be thoroughly understood through years of experience. I mention this because it would not be correct to assume because someone shouts inappropriately, or because someone says 'I cannot see the wood for the trees', that this means they have to be suffering from a *primary* Wood imbalance. It *may* be so, but not necessarily. The above then is a sketch, an outline, so that the methods of acupuncture diagnosis can be better understood.

SEEING

This leads to the third part of the diagnosis, the seeing – which reveals the greatest amount of information. It is perhaps more valuable than any of the other three techniques. First, the practitioner is looking for colours in certain parts of the face. This is not superficial skin colour but more a hue which is present whenever there is an imbalance in any organ in the body, or of any element. It needs skill and experience to be able to discern these colours.

As an example, with our Wood imbalance, a greenish colour can be seen in specific areas of the face. This is the colour that is emanating when either the liver or the gall bladder is malfunctioning. In addition, there are other little hints that together may indicate this imbalance. The person may have an obvious preference for wearing green; or surrounding himself or herself with green. On the other hand he or she may detest green, and wouldn't wear it under any circumstances. Either of these two tendencies, the passion *or* the distaste, may well be indicative of Wood imbalance.

Consider yourself how at one stage in your life you may have craved for a colour and really loved that certain colour; you went, as it were, almost potty over that particular colour. But then, as time passed, this craving diminished. Now you just see that colour in the same light as all the others. You may even dislike it now.

The practitioner will also watch how the patient moves, look at his or her posture, see where there are expressions which may determine 'where the patient is coming from.' He will look very closely at expressions on the face, look at the texture of the hair, and at the skin and the nails. He will note how the patient takes care of him or her self – of their body, of their clothes. All these things can give so much information about attitude.

It is also necessary to observe any defects of function; or scars, physical and mental; how the patient responds to different situations – to meeting a new person, to sorting out appointments, how they talk about themselves.

All of these observations can give information about any elemental imbalance. So, for example, the patient with a Wood imbalance may be wearing green, and showing a dark greenish colour on the face. He may be very rigid and 'woody' in his body structure, generally tense and moving rather jerkily. He may look rather hard despite his smile. His clothes may be scrupulously clean to a degree of fastidiousness. Or he may again, give the impression of being totally and utterly uncared for. He may meet another person rather brightly; but there's a certain aggressive defensiveness about him as he talks, and he may have difficulty in deciding when to make his next appointment. Should it be at this time or that time, this day or another day? Or he may say, 'Oh, I can come at 11.00 o'clock every Monday', and be extremely precise. Or he may even try to dictate when he wants to come. He knows that that is the time that he wants the practitioner to put aside for him and he doesn't want him to give that time to anyone else. He may be expressing all of this aggressively, or apparently with complete absence of anger.

Seeing is of such great importance. So many assume, first of all, that seeing is just something that we do with our physical eye, and by and large, that is what most of us do. It is necessary simply to get us from A to B. We make our decisions primarily on what we see in this cursory way. And yet we are only half-seeing. And when we are sick, we are perhaps not even seeing a quarter of what it is important to see.

The practitioner is trained to look fully into the state of the patient. Is the patient only looking with his physical eye, in a half-hearted way? Is he or she not able to see with the mind's eye? Or, more importantly, is he or she not able to see with the spirit, or the eye of the spirit? Perhaps he or she is just looking at things and evaluating things solely in a material way? Many of us do that. A person may be seen to be not in touch with the overwhelming joy and beauty that is there in so many things, particularly in Nature's own garden.

This faculty can be best evaluated in the way that we see each other. How many of us, to be honest, have made comments that we like this person, or we dislike that person? We are so willing to make that decision just on the basis of what we see superficially. If the face is pleasant, we may well be drawn towards them, and, if they are nicely dressed, again we may be drawn towards them. But, if the face is perhaps not at all pleasant, and they are unkempt and scruffy, we are less likely to be drawn towards them. We may even say disparaging things about them. You see, this is looking only with the physical or unprofessional eye. And the sadness is how much joy and beauty we could otherwise offer to them because really there is that link with God underneath. There is that God, that joy, that beauty and that essential offering within every single person. It can well be that this joy is really more evident in the person who doesn't look so attractive, whose clothes may not be so well cared for. There may be such beauty within such a person that it attracts our attention if we really look.

What a great joy it can be to each of us if we are able to see that essential essence which is there within every human being, and within every living cell, and within every flower, and every blade of grass, and every tree.

The traditional practitioner should, the whole time, be developing his sight to this level so that he can see beneath the surface and is never guilty of making treatment decisions purely on the basis of a physical body and the outward appearance of things.

FEELING

The fourth technique of diagnosis is feeling. Again, there is a tremendous amount of information to be collected here. Feeling does not mean only physically feeling the patient. Whenever you meet someone you can get the feel of him; you sense what sort of a person he is. You can feel his presence in the room, get a sense of his emotional make-up, and also get a sense of his spirit – whether he is a man of great spirit, of great courage, or poor-spirited, very low in confidence, and so on. You feel this, and you can relate to that feeling.

This brings me to the most important 'feeling' procedure of all in traditional Chinese diagnosis – taking of the pulses. Through touch, the traditional practitioner differentiates twelve pulses, six on each wrist. From feeling these pulses, he is able to read the exact state of the vital *Ch'i* energy that is flowing through each of the twelve meridians. He can feel the smallest imbalance in the energy long before it becomes noticeable as a physical symptom. It is possible, only from reading the pulses, to tell almost everything about a patient's state of health. During the examination, the pulses will be taken several times by the practitioner.

In the physical examination, the practitioner will also be feeling the texture and quality of the skin, the temperature of the skin, the temperature of different parts of the body, and the umbilical pulse during abdominal diagnosis. He will be checking the mobility of joints and feeling the spine for misalignments. As he examines the patient in this way, he can also receive a lot of helpful information through watching the patient's reaction to his touch.

The whole of this examination procedure can take two hours or more. By then the practitioner will have collected a lot of information about the state of each of the five elements, and about each of the twelve meridians. He may, by then, have a strong feeling that he knows which one of the elements is the primary one, the one which is the cause of the trouble, the one that is giving rise to the disease. But he must consider other things before coming to his final conclusion.

Before we go on to this, can you say something more about the Chinese method of pulse-taking?

As I have said, the doctor of acupuncture is able to feel twelve different pulses on the two wrists. He feels six on the left wrist – namely the pulses of the heart, the small intestine, the liver, the gall bladder, the kidney and the urinary bladder meridians. And then the six on the right wrist – namely those of the lungs, the colon, the spleen, the stomach, the cirulation-sex and the three-heater meridians.

These twelve pulses are located at specific positions on the wrists. Although the practitioner feels the blood flowing in the radial artery, just as a Western physician does, he is actually assessing the quantity and the quality of the vital *Chi'i* energy that is present in those specific positions along the artery. At each of the twelve positions it is possible to feel the exact state of the *Ch'i* energy within a particular meridian, and hence the state of the organ which it controls. It is the *Ch'i* energy in the liver meridian, for example, that is feeding the liver organ and so, from reading the pulse of the liver meridian, he can tell how the official of the liver meridian is functioning and how the organ itself is functioning.

Many Western-trained doctors who come to train for acupuncture practice find pulse-taking one of the most difficult possibilities to accept. It seems difficult for them to concede that you can read, for example, the condition of the liver, the kidneys and the stomach in what they understand as simply an artery. However, they find in practice, when learning to take these twelve pulses themselves, that they can eventually feel the subtle differences between one position and another. At first they endeavour to explain this variation as being due to the anatomy of the wrist – that the artery feels stronger in one place because it is closer to the surface whilst in another it goes deep, and all sorts of similar explanations. But they become convinced of the actual value of the pulse-taking when they give their first treatment.

After they have read the pulses and planned their treatment, they needle the appropriate point. On re-reading the pulses, they are amazed to find that the pulses have already changed. The pulse they thought was weaker because the artery ran deep now feels as strong as the pulse that they thought was stronger because it was nearer to the surface. They usually have no idea why this pulse change happens but by now they are firmly convinced that it does. After further experience they find, as do all those involved in the practice of traditional Chinese medicine, that the multiple pulses do exist and that they are invaluable in diagnosis and treatment planning; also in ascertaining the efficacy of treatment carried out.

Is it easy to learn to read the twelve pulses?

No, it is not. The reading of the pulses takes a great deal of practice. It requires much work to develop the sensitivity of the fingertips. The true master of pulse-taking, who has many, many years of experience, is able to feel twenty-eight different qualities within each of the twelve pulses. From these readings, he is able to tell what has been, what is, and what will be, as far as the patient's health of body, mind and spirit is concerned.

When you spoke about 'asking', you mentioned that a patient may feel better or worse at a particular time of day. Can you say why this is?

I spoke earlier of the Chinese people observing the cycles of night and day, and their seeing that the quality of energy changed with the sun's rising in the sky, and with the sun's sinking away into the following night time. With keen observation they saw that likewise each of the twelve meridians has a peak time of activity and one of passiveness in this twenty-four hour cycle. The wave of peak energy moved from one meridian into the next in a continuous cycle around the body throughout the day and night.

So, for example, they found that the energy in the gall bladder meridian peaked from eleven o'clock at night until one o'clock in the morning, and the liver peaked from one o'clock in the morning till three o'clock in the morning, and so on round the cycle of twelve meridians. This is invaluable knowledge in diagnosis. For example, a person may say, 'I am never able to go to sleep until three o'clock in the morning.' This may arouse suspicion about the Wood element. It sounds as if the gall bladder and the liver officials are too active before that time to allow the patient to fall asleep. Or another person may say he wakes up at one o'clock in the morning, or three o'clock in the morning, with a blinding headache. From the times given for intensification of pain, or worsening of discomfort, and so on, the practitioner can very often have attention drawn to a specific organ.

The opposite to the peak time in the twenty-four hour cycle is the period when the meridian is resting. A person may say 'I get terribly low and depressed in the middle of the day. It starts about eleven o'clock in the morning.' This may well be pointing to the fact that the body cannot cope when the energy in one of the Wood meridians is at its very lowest.

The energy on earth follows this same pattern of peaks and lows, and it is traditionally referred to by the Chinese as the

Law of Midday and Midnight. This law, again, is much more complicated than is suggested in the brief description given above, but I am giving it to you in outline to show how time of day is related to certain organs. Again, I advise that you do not however start making self-diagnosis. The fact that a pain may intensify, or get better, between one o'clock and three o'clock in the morning does not necessarily mean that the cause is from the liver; it could be coming from any other organ but having an effect through the liver.

Having done this initial examination, what other things does a practitioner consider in order to decide which was the first meridian to become out of balance, or the one that caused the disease?

You will remember we also looked earlier at the cycle of the seasons; for example, how spring moves into summer. I pointed out that we can view this seasonal change as Wood becoming Fire; or it would be better to say, Wood creating Fire. Thus, if the patient is exhibiting many symptoms of Wood imbalance, we would expect there to be some signs of trouble in the Fire element too. A weak Wood energy is not going to create a very strong Fire energy. So, we notice that our patient is showing some signs of a Fire imabalance. He seems to have a lack of joy, or he is craving for sunshine, or warmth, or heat. But we can still say that this is probably due to a primary Wood energy imbalance.

But supposing we also find that our patient has problems in the Earth element. For example, he is eating too many sweet things – an appetite which he just cannot control – although he may be very careful about diet in other respects. I suggested earlier that such a person may be rather rigid and tight. He reacts very strongly when offered sympathy over his problems, or his symptoms; he dislikes this sympathy and rejects it; he becomes even more rigid. Could these Earth symptoms make sense? And the answer is that they could.

The Chinese saw, from observing the seasons, that there is a cycle of control. A farmer will tell you that his harvest of late summer can be no better than was made possible by the kind of spring that year. How much blossom was there? Did it get pollinated? Was it a cold spring? Thus the spring, in a sense, can be seen to exert an influence over late summer. Similarly, this process whereby the effects in one season influence succeeding seasons applies all through the cycle.

If we replace the seasons with the elements of the same quality of *Ch'i* energy (see diagram opposite), then we can see that Wood controls Earth, and so on round the cycle.

Thus, if the Wood energy is in trouble, we can expect the Earth energy to become imbalanced. It's not being adequately controlled. So, although the patient is showing signs of an imbalance in both the Earth energy and the Wood energy, it makes sense for us to think that the primary imbalance may be in the Wood energy.

This brings me to an extraordinary piece of observation, made by the Chinese, that has far-reaching effects both in diagnosis and in treatment. Let us go back to the patient whom I have described as having signs of primary imbalance in the Wood energy. That is to say, that imbalance there is really more noticeable than in any of the other elements. Where does this Wood energy come from? As I have shown on the diagram, it has been created from the preceding element. Wood is dependent upon the Water element. Or we could say that the Water element is the mother of the Wood energy.

When describing these terms it seems as though we are now speculating and trying to illustrate and substantiate theories. But the Chinese looked at the mother breast-feeding her baby and saw her natural love and concern for her child. They saw that if the mother became ill, she was perhaps no longer able to produce enough milk for her child; or the milk perhaps became poor in quality. So the little baby became more and more hungry, and thus cried and cried. The mother, of course, would become greatly distressed. Whilst ill, maybe others tried to feed the baby; but the baby cried even more. It only wanted its mother's breast and its mother's love and its mother's milk.

If we look casually at such a scene, we might first think that it is the child, making such cries of distress, who is ill and needing treatment. But we would be wrong. What is really

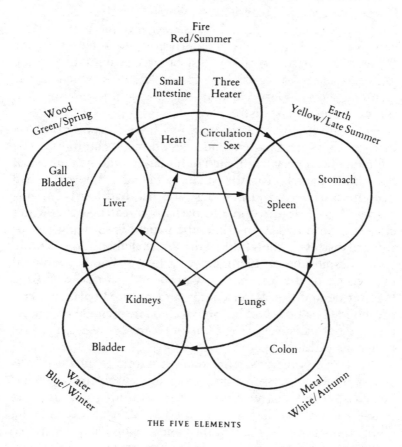

THE FIVE ELEMENTS

needed in this situation is to do everything possible to restore the mother to health. Once she is well, she will then be able to feed her baby with the right quality and the right volume of milk, and give the child that tender loving care that only a mother can give. Then, of course, the baby will stop crying.

So, if we come back now to the patient, and we see that the Wood energy is in great distress, we ask ourselves if this is the 'child crying in distress', because 'its mother is no longer capable of feeding it'. We would need to look closely at the Water element to see if it is just bravely struggling to keep going in order to do its best for its 'child' – which, is the element Wood. Here we may find the solution – find that which is causing the distress.

For example, the practitioner may note, in taking the case history, that such a patient had a very difficult childhood. The child had been very frightened of his father who had punished the child severely for the smallest failings. The child had become introvert, and nervous, and had had terrible night-mares. This fear early in life perhaps threatened the Water element. So now, as an adult, the patient is showing symp-toms of distress in the 'child' of the Water element – the Wood.

So, despite the problem showing in the Wood, we would need to go to the 'mother' – Water – and get that well first. Having treated the Water energy and restored balance there, the 'child – Wood – will become well on its own. The Chinese referred to this aspect of the *Shen* (or creative) cycle, as the Law of Mother/Child.

I will give you an example demonstrating the value of this Law. Suppose a person is suffering from a problem which has been diagnosed by a Western doctor as a heart condition – let us say tachycardia. The patient is taking drugs for this. But a Chinese doctor – diagnosing the patient in his terms – may see that although there are signs of the Fire energy, or the heart, being in great trouble, the problem really lies in the 'mother', the Wood energy. So it would be the Wood energy that would be treated – which, in terms of the organs, would mean helping the liver and the gall bladder.

The liver meridian is the 'mother of the heart', so that as the liver is treated, then tachycardia, or any other heart symptoms would disappear. The tragedy can be that, if the heart only is continually treated, the condition is palliated but the patient never really gets better.

From what you say it seems that it is quite a complicated procedure diagnosing which meridian has first collapsed under stress. Can this be done by the end of the first examination?

Frequently the practitioner will know which is the primary meridian needing help – or the causative factor of the disease – by the end of the initial consultation. But it would be better to say that, after the consultation which may take some two hours, all the information is carefully considered by the practitioner. He or she may spend considerable time going through this procedure before clarifying and confirming the causative factor, or the cause of the disease. This is why you will rarely be treated at the end of the initial examination. The practitioner needs to work on all this information for some while before confirming the causative factor of disease and proceeding to treat.

What could a patient expect to be told after the examination?

This will vary from practitioner to practitioner, and from patient to patient. Certainly, as I have already indicated, the patient should not expect a diagnosis in Western terms. After the consultation and preliminary work on the case notes, the practitioner will often be willing to share his finding and he will usually speak of the cause of the energy imbalance and the cause of the disease in acupuncture terms.

He will usually try to explain what he is hoping to achieve, and stage by stage during the treatment, should the patient so desire, he will explain what is happening. We feel this is of the utmost importance. After all, it is your body, your mind and your spirit that we are hoping to restore to balance. In so doing, it is only right that you should know as much as possible about what is going on. In this respect we find that patients themselves can assist and co-operate with the treatment if they understand what we are trying to achieve.

31

Is it difficult to learn this method of diagnosis – to be able to see the different elements manifesting in a person, to be able to see the colour in the face, to hear the sound of the voice, to smell the odour, to recognise inappropriate emotions, and to read the pulses?

It is certainly more difficult than may be thought at first. The fact is that we cannot see, we cannot hear, we cannot smell and we cannot feel. Perhaps, to be fair, I should say we only use a fraction of our capacity in these spheres. In case the reader may at first take exception to this statement, I will explain what I mean.

One of the reasons it takes so long to become proficient in traditional Chinese acupuncture is that people have usually failed to develop the senses that God gave them when they were born. Instead of developing these senses, they have been ignored – and in some cases abused – until they have become dull, and need to be re-trained.

For example, our vision is very limited. We only see what we choose to see in order to achieve our aims – which, indeed, are often as limited as our vision. Supposing we leave home in the morning to go shopping or to work, and on the way we pass a tree in blossom, or a flower bed surrounded by lawn, or we look out over a field, and we pass some people. A friend may ask us later 'Did you see that beautiful tree in blossom?' or, 'Did you see that flowerbed?' And we reply, 'Yes, I saw it. It was beautiful.' Or they may say 'Did you see Mary, or John?' and we reply, 'Yes, I saw them on the way to work,' or 'I saw them on the way to the shops'. We may even comment on Mary's dress or on what John was doing. I regret this is indicative of the casual and superficial way the average person in the Western world uses that most precious gift of sight.

If we were really to look at one of the flowers in the flower-bed and see it for what it really is, we would see something of indescribable majesty and beauty; and we would almost feel the life and the vibration coming from that flower. It is something that Nature has created for all of us to enjoy. When holding the flower in our hand, and seeing it not just with a cursory glance as we did before, but looking into the structure and the texture and the colours and the shape, we find we can almost see it, not just with the physical eye, but with the mind's eye. Just for a moment we may even glimpse it with the eye of the spirit.

Supposing also, we were to look closely into the tree in blossom, we would notice and appreciate the majesty and the wonder of that tree; and we would see how different that tree is from every other tree in the whole of the world. There are no two trees the same; there are no two blades of grass the same; there are no two flowers the same; and there are no two people the same. If we could spare the time to see that tree as it is – a unique and individual wonder created by nature – and if we could look at that tree not with a cursory glance but with time to see it with our physical eye, our mind's eye and our spirit eye, then we could be overcome by the tremendous beauty that is there for all to see. Yet we don't find the time. We just pass these things as we go from point A to B. And we say 'Yes, I saw that flower, I saw that grass, I saw that tree'. That is what I mean when I say our vision is limited.

When we say things like 'I do see this, I did see that', we are in fact making full claim on what we have seen only with a degree of our physical sight – we see perhaps only one fifth of what is really there to be seen.

This is, of course, and surely more importantly, just as applicable in how we see human beings. We may even be repulsed by someone just because of the way they are dressed. But if we stopped, and we afforded the time with each in- dividual, we would see again the unique beauty and the God that is within every living human person. This would give us a true appreciation of our fellow humans – of our own brothers and sisters. Yet how often we make judgements and decisions in the light of what we have only partially seen with our physical eye. And it is overcoming this dull habit that makes training in traditional Chinese acupuncture difficult.

What I have said about sight is equally applicable to hearing. As a rule we only hear what we want to hear, and we shut out what we do not wish to hear. We may hear the words them- selves, but we don't stop to hear the sound in the words, or listen to the expression behind them – those features that come from a deeper source within the person.

The same limitation can certainly be said of our sense of smell and our sense of touch. Yet do we recall loving parents explaining these things to children and encouraging them to use these gifts to a maximum?

If they did so, the result would be happier, more contented children. But no. Unfortunately, we tend to just accept these gifts as our right, and instead of developing them and using them fully, we abuse them and neglect them – perhaps too blinded in pursuit of academic learning, status, position, a better job. It is as if we have cast aside the beauty of the seasons and the quality of life in order to grasp possessions in the material world and follow selfish pursuits. It is as if we have a glass of fresh spring water to drink, and yet choose to drink from a stagnant pond.

I would like to add here that I believe there is a limit to what any man or woman can teach you. Our truest and most profound teacher is Nature herself. Nature is there before us to teach us about life so that we may fully develop within ourselves. We need to be open-minded, restore our senses and become sensitive to Nature's wisdom. Consider a child – one that has not yet been misguided or manipulated, or conditioned to believe in the material ends in pursuit of which most people live today. There you will see a beauty, a simplicity of heart and sensitivity beyond comprehension.

A baby can virtually 'see' his mother, even if she is out of range of his physical eyes. A baby can feel the presence of his mother even though she may be out of sight. A baby can just touch, and recognise from touch alone, whether the person is familiar or not – and only because the child is using his God-given senses in order to find his or her way in this world. Each of us had this capacity once.

This is the kind of sensitivity needed by the acupuncture practitioner. Many years of hard work are required to regain it. Only then will he or she be able to recognise accurately the distress signals from the body, mind and spirit, and be able to interpret and utilize the natural laws which govern traditional Chinese medicine.

So to return to the question. It is difficult for a Western trainee to learn to be able to detect and read correctly the

34

meaning of the signals given by a person's body, mind and spirit – by the elements that are in trouble. In order to do so, he or she has to develop his or her awareness. The diagnosis becomes easier for the practitioner the more he or she develops his or her own natural gifts.

Will the acupuncturist carry out any of the common Western diagnostic procedures as well?

He will carry out some of them. We are, after all, living in Western-conditioned communities, and it is thus sensible to make some use of the valuable information that can be gained from Western medical tests. Such procedures are taught in many colleges by Western-trained doctors and tutors from Western hospitals and students are examined in these subjects.

A master of acupuncture – who has had, say, thirty or forty years' experience – would not need to incorporate any Western procedures in his diagnosis in order to reach his conclusions. Until such proficiency is achieved, however, practitioners make use of some of the Western procedures and incorporate them in the initial examination. This is done to confirm what has been found from the traditional diagnosis. Procedures such as taking blood pressure and listening to the heart and the lungs with a stethoscope are useful contributions to diagnosis. Other diagnostic techniques – such as electro-cardiograms and urine analysis – may also be employed. But, fundamentally, the physical examination will be made in terms of traditional Chinese medicine.

5 The Use of Needles

Is anything in or on the needles inserted during acupuncture treatment?

If you are going to a traditionally trained acupuncturist, then no drugs of any kind are injected, no electrical charge or current is applied, and nothing is placed on or in the needles.

What are the needles like?

They are usually of stainless steel, not much thicker than a human hair. They are solid – not hollow like needles used for injections in Western medical practice.

Does the needle hurt?

It is hard to describe the sensation felt. One person will experience the effect of the needle differently from another. Some people find them a little painful, but only momentarily. Usually nothing is felt as the needle penetrates the skin but there will be some sensation as the needle reaches the subcutaneous acupuncture point. This can be a feeling of numbness, or an ache, or an 'alive' sensation, or a sort of sharpness. It is certainly a lot less painful than the sensation when accidentally punctured by a needle or pin. Some people seem to feel hardly anything at all.

Does insertion of an acupuncture needle compare, in terms of pain,
with an injection in Western medical practice?

There is really no comparison. Many people imagine injection
with a hypodermic syringe when you mention acupuncture. But
it is *far less* unpleasant. There are often occasions when a patient can
be quite unaware that the acupuncture needle has been inserted.

Do the needles vary in length? And are there different types?

Yes, the most common needles vary in length from half-an-
inch to one-and-a-half inches. There are different types of
needle and they are used according to the preference of the
practitioner (although certain needles have particular functions,
e.g., those used in conjunction with moxa treatment (see p.41).

To what depth are the needles inserted?

The depth of the insertion of the needle varies considerably.
Usually needles are inserted just below the skin surface since
most acupuncture points lie just under it. But some needles
need to penetrate to a depth from a quarter-of-an-inch to as
much as one-and-a-half to two inches, depending on the appropriate acupuncture points being used. The depth is also
affected by the amount of fat carried by the patient.

But do not assume that the deeper the insertion the more the
patient will feel. The patient will feel no more discomfort from
a needle inserted three inches below the skin as that from a
needle inserted just below the skin. Nothing is felt until the
needle acts upon the acupuncture point.

Is the needle manipulated after the insertion?

This depends on the effect desired. A subtle manipulation is
always employed. This is a very technical matter – but the
patient is often unaware of needle manipulation since the entire
procedure is smooth-flowing, subtle and very gentle.

How many needles are commonly used?

This varies from one patient to another, and upon the required treatment. Usually two to six needles are used in one treatment. But there are occasions when a practitioner will need to use more. I think perhaps this question is often asked because of articles which have been published in magazines – showing someone lying prostrate with perhaps as many as forty or fifty needles inserted. This quantity would be unnecessary in traditional practice.

The number of needles used is not an indication of the competence of the practitioner or the value of the treatment. More needles do not mean better treatment. You will never be punctured like a pepper pot!

Into which part of the body does the acupuncturist insert the needles?

As I explained earlier, each meridian has a specific pathway in the body. It passes through the organ which gives the meridian its name. Each meridian has a superficial pathway close to the surface of the skin and it is here that the acupuncture points are located. The most frequently used points lie on the lower parts of the legs, the feet, the forearms and the hands. There are, however, other points, over the whole body, that are also often used.

This wide range of points is appropriate because, in traditional acupuncture, one is not concerned with treating regional symptoms. The parts of the body into which needles are inserted often bear no relation to the site of the symptoms. But the particular points which command the general energy flow of the entire meridian lie in the forearms and the hands, and the lower legs and the feet. Therefore these are the points that are most commonly used.

Does the patient bleed very much?

The needle insertion points will not bleed. In ninety-nine out of every hundred insertions there will be no blood-letting whatsoever. However, the needle may prick a superficial capillary lying near to the acupuncture point; that may cause a little bleeding or bruising. This would be very unusual. And there are very rare occasions when – as the Chinese say – the blood has 'got into the meridian' and blocked it. On these occasions a practitioner may, purposely, bleed a point. The result would be only one or two, at the most three, drops of blood; and then the bleeding would cease.

Can a needle ever break or bend during treatment?

A needle may sometimes bend slightly if the patient moves vigorously as, or after, the needle has been inserted. Breakage or snapping off of the needle is impossible if the practitioner uses the best quality needles. Every adequately-trained practitioner will know the importance of using the best quality needles. These needles are diamond–drawn stainless steel with no joint betwen the handle and the shaft. Such needles are so pliable that they can be tied into a knot without breaking. Thus it should be impossible for them to break during treatment.

Are the needles only made in China? Does their effect depend on the material used?

Needles are manufactured in many countries throughout the world, I personally use hand–made Chinese needles.

You may have heard of gold and silver needles being used for certain effects. This idea has probably arisen from mistakes made in the translation of old Chinese texts. The needles themselves were then made of the finest materials but they were mounted on either gold or silver handles according to whether they were to be used for treating the mandarin classes or lower classes. In the West, there is a tendency to attach too much importance to the value of the needle itself. The effect of the treatment is not due to the type of metal or the value of the material of which the needle is made. In China, acupuncture was practised long before metal needles were invented; they then used needles of bone or stone.

Are the needles sterilized before treatment?

Yes. This is of paramount importance. There is a risk, otherwise, of transferring viral or bacterial infection.

The needles are sterilized before every insertion. In many cases the practitioner will keep particular needles for a particular patient – to be used with that patient alone.

Hygienically-acceptable methods of sterilization vary from area to area, and every properly trained practitioner must comply with the regulations laid down by the health authority. These vary slightly from area to area. Such regulations include sterilization by autoclaving, boiling and hot air. The harshness of such methods eventually causes deterioration of needle quality so each needle is checked for barbs, pitting and bluntness after each sterilization. Needles are thrown away at the first sign of any deterioration.

It is also standard practice to wipe the patient's skin with a sterilizing fluid before each insertion of a needle. At all times, sterilization procedure is paramount in the practitioner's mind. In the twenty-one years of the College of Traditional Chinese Acupuncture's history, I cannot recall a single case where a graduate practitioner has been found negligent in this very important matter. There has never been a case of hepatitis or transferred infection due to negligence by a graduate of this College. This, I think, testifies to the tremendous emphasis placed on this aspect of practice by the properly-trained practitioner of traditional acupuncture.

6   The Use of Moxa and
Other Treatments

Does the practitioner use any treatment other than needles?

Yes; and in some cases no needles at all are used. A special form
of massage may be used on the acupuncture points and sometimes a system of Chinese osteopathy is practised. Also the
points may be heated in various ways.

How is this heat applied to acupuncture points?

The commonest way is for a small cone of moxa to be placed
on the point and ignited. Moxa is made from the stripped and
dried leaves of a Chinese mugwort-like herb called *artemisia
vulgaris latiflora*. It is like a brown-coloured wool in appearance. The acupuncture point is greatly affected by the heat.
Usually, three to five cones are used in succession on each
acupuncture point, but sometimes there may be more. And
the moxa may occasionally be burnt on a bed of garlic, ginger
or salt to produce special effects.

Alternatively, a point or area of the skin may be heated less
directly by using a large, burning moxa stick, three-quarters
of an inch to one-and-a-half inches in diameter. This is passed
backwards and forwards over the skin, just close enough to
give a comfortable heat.

Does the moxa ever burn the skin?

No. After the tip of the moxa cone is ignited, it slowly burns down. The practitioner asks the patient to say when sufficient heat is felt, and as soon as that happens, the remaining moxa is removed. It is not left on the skin long enough to cause a burn and therefore, if the treatment is carried out correctly, there is no danger of scarring.

What is the difference in effect between using moxa and using needles?

Moxa has a warming, nourishing effect upon the *Ch'i* energy, and, where this effect is most appropriate – depending on the patient or the nature of the imbalance – it may be used instead of needles. But usually both are used, the moxa first, and then the needle. Or the moxa may be placed on the head of a special needle and ignited, and a gentle heat is carried to the point that way.

Where appropriate – if the patient has a real fear of needles, or sometimes in the case of children – it may be possible to use moxa and massage alone, not using needles at all.

You mention a form of massage. I have seen articles in newspapers which said that there are certain points which one can rub oneself to relieve certain symptoms. I take it that this is not proper acupuncture?

No. This practice can be regarded as a form of 'local–doctor' (see p.69–72) or symptomatic acupuncture. Massaging points can result in suppression of symptoms. But, whilst the symptoms are being palliated, the disease may be worsening at a deeper level. To put this into perspective, however, if one were to have just an *occasional* headache, or perhaps a tooth-ache, or a tummy ache, then massaging certain points can certainly bring helpful and welcome relief. But if one were plagued with *continual* headaches or *continual* tummy aches, or whatever, then each relief would surely be a suppression. So, in one instance, as temporary first-aid, the massage is valuable, but as a repeated treatment for recurring and persistent symptoms, it is extremely dangerous. For example, if someone were getting continual headaches – perhaps through a liver imbalance

– massaging certain points on the body may alleviate the headaches but it does nothing whatsoever to deal with the *cause* of the headache – the imbalance or malfunction of the liver or its associated energies.

A traditional acupuncturist would ascertain the cause of the headaches, i.e. the liver, and would endeavour to balance and harmonize the energy of the liver. The headaches would disappear and would not then return, unless of course the patient was in some way creating a situation in his or her life which made it impossible for the liver meridian to maintain the balance. For example, if the patient were in the habit of drinking excessive amounts of alcohol or taking excessive amounts of drugs.

7 Types of Illness Helped by Acupuncture

I hesitate a little at the title of this chapter because it suggests that the acupuncturist focuses on particular labelled illnesses instead of looking at the state of the whole person. What we call a certain illness is really an indication of an underlying energy imbalance. Thus, it is really inappropriate for an acupuncturist to speak of treating a labelled disease. Because we are all unique individuals, so we will each have a different reason for a labelled disease manifesting as it does. The symptoms may manifest in the same way but the underlying cause will be different.

To assume that the cause of a certain common complaint – called, say, 'migraine' – is exactly the same in all sufferers from a particular kind of headache is to ignore the unique nature and constitution of each person. This is contrary to common sense and the evidence, let alone Chinese medical thinking. It makes a mockery of Nature's infinite variety.

Having said that, there are certain questions that can be answered in the terms of particular illnesses. But it must be borne in mind that in every case referred to a traditional acupuncturist, he or she will be considering the person as a whole – as a unique body, mind and spirit – and not just in those limited, common terms.

I suppose what most people are saying, when they ask 'Can you cure migraine?' or 'Can you cure depression?' is 'Have you had success with conditions similar to mine?' (It is in this sense that they use the labels.) But, to be honest, the practitioner cannot be certain whether a patient will or will not benefit until he has carried out the traditional examination and has seen how the patient responds to the first few treatments.

May disease have gone too far for acupuncture to be able to help?

A time does come when disease has gone beyond the reach of effective treatment, and the sufferer is beyond human help. The practitioner would know after a few treatments if this were the case and would be morally bound to tell the patient so. Nevertheless, acupuncture treatment could still then be used to help ease pain. This is one of the rare occasions when the practitioner could legitimately resort to 'local-doctor' or analgesia treatment – to make the patient as comfortable as possible for the remainder of his or her life. But this must only be done with the understanding and the consent of the patient after the practitioner has honestly explained the situation.

In what circumstances would you definitely not recommend acupuncture treatment?

I would not recommend acupuncture treatment in emergencies resulting from accident or advanced diseases – where immediate surgical or medical treatment is needed to save the patient's life. And there are the terminal cases mentioned above, where the patient is beyond human help (other than relief of pain and suffering).

There are also cases where a decision to treat or not to treat is difficult to reach. Consequently, in every case, after examining the patient, I ask myself whether or not acupuncture really is the best form of treatment for him or her. For a number of reasons it might be better to recommend treatment by orthodox medicine – by surgery, or whatever. In all cases of doubt, my guideline is to ask myself what I would recommend if, for instance, the patient were my wife, my son or my daughter.

Many people who are chronically ill are constantly under drugs – for various reasons, including relief of pain. Does this make treatment with acupuncture more difficult?

It certainly does not make the practitioner's task any easier. Drugs may bring great relief to sufferers but, in the long run, they can harm the body and they introduce something further for it to cope with. Rather than rid the patient of the disease, they tend to suppress it and make it go deeper. And then there may be additional effects whereby further symptoms result from the drugs themselves, adding to the original complaint for which the patient is seeking relief.

Nevertheless, having said that, one needs to allow relief and afford a safeguard to the patient, without any ill effects. This depends on the individual, on the drug and on the dosage.

A healthy body itself makes all the 'drugs' that it needs to fight diseases, repair damage, and keep itself in balance; a sick body does not. Acupuncture aims to restore and maintain the body's own ability to produce the necessary enzymes and secretions, insulin, pepsin, adrenalin, cortisone, hydrochloric acid and the like.

Does this mean that acupuncture can cure certain deficiency diseases?

In many cases, deficiency diseases, if we wish to use that term, respond well to acupuncture treatment. In the West we tend to think that if a patient is deficient in a substance we can cure him or her by giving doses of the substance concerned. For example, we give iron (for anaemia), insulin (for diabetes), vitamins, calcium, hormones, and so on. The introduction of these substances does not correct the deficiency permanently; it only keeps the body going. Acupuncture aims to correct the *cause* of the deficiency, thus enabling the body either to produce the necessary substance itself or enabling it to extract what it requires from the normal balanced diet. But again, it should be added, acupuncture is successful in certain circumstances; in other circumstances, it is not.

Can acupuncture help in the case of addiction: drugs, alcohol or smoking?

Yes, it can. A person who is perfectly healthy in body, mind and spirit does not need the comfort, help or stimulus of drugs or alcohol. Addiction to any of these is a sign of insecurity, stress or strain, all of which are difficult to avoid in modern living. Acupuncture can temporarily correct the energy imbalance that has arisen as a result but a permanent cure depends upon the removal or resolution of the stresses that caused the addiction.

To go beyond just answering the question as simply as that, I feel that one needs to take a balanced look at these tendencies to addiction. It is so easy to decry drugs, alcohol and smoking, and, whilst I have no desire to take sides, I feel that a sense of proportion and tolerance would perhaps permit a growth within ourselves of the ability to look at all of these things more rationally and compassionately – rather than hastily taking a biased, prejudiced and hostile view.

To illustrate what I am trying to convey, let me first take the case of smoking. One has seen in recent years a vast amount of publicity directed towards the dangers of smoking and I don't really think anyone, smoker or non-smoker, could deny much that is presented against the practice, i.e. the incidence of lung diseases, of cardiac conditions, the vast amount of money spent in hospital care of such people, and so on. It becomes very easy to condemn smokers as social outcasts, as idiots who get their just desserts. How many times have I heard this point laboured by someone who is holding a glass of whisky in his hand!

Supposing we consider alcohol in the same way – we would see the vast number of people who suffer from diseases of the liver and the kidneys, and, perhaps more important, the mental diseases that are brought on by the abuse of alcohol. Here again we would have to note the great number of beds occupied in hospitals, and the time and money spent on caring for such people, whom we could say, again, are getting their just desserts.

But why stop there? The same sort of comments could be made about the takers of drugs, even those that are prescribed by medical practitioners. Here we would find many cases of dependence after repeat prescriptions, vast amounts of over-the-counter drugs consumed without doctor supervision – all at enormous expense. Here again, one could point out the large number of people taking up hospital beds with drug-related side-effects and illnesses. To go a stage further, even in the habit of eating we can find addiction. People addicted to food tend to become excessively overweight. And the same consequences happen again – ill-health and illness as a result of the conditions brought about by excessive eating. (The same applies to the opposite – people who make themselves ill through excessive dieting.) These again become a drain upon our medical and hospital resources.

So, if we are going to take sides against the smoker, we must also, in fairness, conduct the offensive against drinking, against drug-dependence, and against over-eating. 'Those who live in glass houses shouldn't throw stones!'

Now to return to the question.

Anyone who smokes excessively, drinks excessively, takes drugs excessively, or eats to excess is, in my view, a sick person. Something is driving them towards this excess. The habit provides some sort of comfort or solace; perhaps it gives a degree of escape from the realities of day-to-day problems, which they are otherwise unable to deal with. Traditional Chinese acupuncture can and does work to remedy these forms of addiction. It can create a better balance and harmony within the body, mind and spirit; then the need for these excesses diminishes.

I see nothing wrong whatsoever in anyone having an occasional drink or an occasional smoke; or occasionally eating junk food or taking a drug (when properly prescribed). A degree of tolerance is needed for balance and harmony. And it is towards achieving this easy balance that the practitioner of traditional Chinese acupuncture will be working with his or her patient.

Can acupuncture be used during pregnancy?

Yes, it can; but it should be administered only by a highly qualified practitioner with long experience. Such a practitioner can safely treat many different illnesses while the patient is pregnant. Apart from any illness, a skilled practitioner can also help promote a healthy pregnancy. By that, I mean one free from morning sickness, overweight problems, depression and so on. In the final month of pregnancy, treatment often facilitates an easier and natural birth.

It is also possible to give acupuncture analgesia during childbirth. The skilled traditional acupuncturist can do this with complete safety since he is trained to be continually aware of the exact state of the mother's energy.

The reason for caution when treating a pregnant woman is due to the fact that whilst treating the mother, the unborn child is being influenced and treated also. This is why I emphasize that its practice needs to be undertaken only by highly qualified practitioners with long experience.

Can acupuncture be used for birth control and abortion?

In some Eastern countries, acupuncture has been used for both birth control and abortion. But such practice would never be undertaken by a qualified practitioner of traditional Chinese acupuncture who has been trained at my College, for various reasons. It would not only be a violation of our code of ethics but it would also be a violation of the natural laws which govern this system of medicine.

Does acupuncture aid the healing of broken bones?

Yes. The patient still needs to have the bones set in the usual way, but acpuncture can and does assist and speed up the healing process. I have attended many cases where it has been possible for casts to be removed some three weeks before they would ordinarily have been due to be taken off.

One of the most successful combinations of modern medicine and traditional Chinese acupuncture has taken place in this field in China. The Chinese claim to have shortened considerably the time taken to heal a fracture by dispensing with the plaster cast and using thin splints instead. While holding the bone firmly in position, the splits allow a certain degree of movement in the neighbouring area. Then, acupuncture treatment, by bringing energy to the area, helps to keep all the normal processes of that area of the body functioning to their optimum, so leading to rapid healing.

Is acupuncture used to treat tumours?

As I have pointed out, the traditional Chinese acupuncturist does not treat named symptoms, and 'tumour' would come into this category. There are many cases recorded where tumours have disappeared or have shrunk considerably during treatment; but there are others where the treatment has had no effect whatsoever. So much depends upon the causative factor of the disease, and how far it has advanced.

What about afflictions like hay fever, other allergies or insomnia? Can acupuncture help?

'Hay fever', 'allergies' and 'insomnia' are, again the names of symptoms. The causes of allergies and insomnia are numerous. Such afflictions can result from tension, worry, fear, depression, grief and a host of other mental states; or they can result from organic malfunction; or, in many cases, they arise from a combination of mental and organic factors. Hay fever, insomnia and other allergies will clear up as the energy of the patient is brought into balance.

Does this mean that mental illnesses come within the scope of acupuncture?

Yes, indeed. I cannot stress too strongly that the practitioner of traditional acupuncture always views the body, mind and spirit as a whole. I wish to emphasize that he does not view them as separate and divided. All physical disorders will cause an imbalance in the mental outlook; this may manifest as depression, anger, sadness, or the like. Also, all mental disturbances will cause some reaction in the physical body; for example, sickness, insomnia, lack of appetite, weariness or aching limbs. It is not possible to have a physical illness on its own, or a mental disorder on its own.

Any imbalance in a person must manifest itself both in the physical body and the mental 'body': two parts of the whole. The spirit may also be affected, of course. Most people can tolerate physical pain to a degree; it is the mental anguish that so many people live with which is unbearable. And when the spirit is badly affected, the person sees no point in continuing to live.

All treatments aim to restore the harmony of the body, the mind and the spirit. So the physical and mental aspects of a person are treated together; and as one improves so does the other.

We hear a lot these days about many illnesses being psychosomatic. You would not completely agree with that, then?

I would direct attention again to the continuous interaction between the body, the mind and the spirit. Suppose a person is suffering from acute depression. This could be the effect of either mental difficulties or of a particular physical disorder – for example, malfunction of the kidneys or the bladder, or of any one or perhaps more of the body's organs. Or it could be due to the person's spirit. Before treatment is given, it is extremely important to diagnose accurately where the cause of the illness lies – in body, mind or spirit.

A patient came to me to be treated for lumbago. When she was better and had finished treatment, her husband came to thank me. He did not thank me for curing her lumbago but for making his life so much happier. He said his wife had previously been so irritable that she had become very difficult to live with. He had had no idea when he offered to pay for her treatment that it was going to make such a change in her whole outlook. She had become a happy, cheerful person again, and, to use his words, they were once again 'like two children'.

It seems that Western medicine does not always appreciate the effect that a physical disorder has on the mental state of a person. (It is gratifying that much more attention is being paid to it nowadays). Each main organ and function has its counterpart in the mind and the spirit. Disorder in the working of each main organ and function has a particular and different effect on the mental state of a person, and his or her spirit. Observation of these different states actually helps the practitioner to determine the source of disorder in the physical body.

Will acupuncture benefit someone who is very sceptical about it?

Yes, certainly. The healing process will not be affected in any way by a patient's sceptical attitude.

However, there may be other factors which will affect the process. A person may, for example, be determined to continue to lead a way of life which will hinder his or her progress. (This in itself would be another sign of sickness). But as treatment proceeds, we would hope to see such a person's attitude and lifestyle change and become more balanced, thus eliminating the hindrance to progress.

8   The Treatment

How many treatments are usually necessary?

This varies considerably from person to person. One cannot be guided by the experience of other patients. Some patients may need less than eight treatments, others may need as many as eighty. A lot depends on the severity of the disease, and how long the patient has suffered from it. What drugs have been, or are being taken – among a host of other factors – can affect speed of progress.

One hears of the occasional 'miracle cure' by acupuncture, when a chronic condition of very long standing has responded to acupuncture so rapidly that the patient is well perhaps after only two or three treatments; but this is very rare. When an illness has become deeply seated, it is to be expected that it will take a long time to rectify. Much patience and work will be needed.

How frequent are the treatments?

This also varies. On average, treatments are given perhaps twice a week for the first two or three weeks, and then once a week. As the patient improves, the visits will be reduced – perhaps to once every two weeks, then once a month.

Will the benefits from the treatment be lasting, or must there be follow up treatments after a few months, or a year or so?

This largely depends on the patient. Follow-up treatments should not be necessary if the patient is living sensibly with moderate diet and habits, and is able to avoid the undue stresses and strains. But if the patient returns to the same conditions and lifestyle that caused the original trouble, the illness will probably recur and more treatments will be necessary.

As a rule, people adopt a sensible attitude. They return to the clinic perhaps once every few months, at the change of each season, for example; or perhaps just once or twice a year for a check up. The practitioner then is able to tell from the pulses if anything is going wrong in the body, the mind or the spirit long before it manifests itself symptomatically. After all, traditional Chinese acupuncture was primarily intended as a preventative system of medicine, and only secondarily as a system of medicine to be used after manifestation of disease.

What does the initial consultation and treatment cost?

It is extremely difficult to give an indication of cost as it will vary from practitioner to practitioner, and according to the facilities that are available. But the charges will be roughly in line with those of other holistic medical practitioners in private practice.

How long does a treatment take?

On average, a treatment takes about one half to three-quarters of an hour, although it should be said that many treatments can take an hour, or even more. The time taken to give the treatment is not the main criterion. The practitioner will have in mind changes that he or she would like to see taking place in the patient during the course of the treatment. As a rule, the patient will not therefore be permitted to leave until those results have been achieved. Sometimes a patient responds wonderfully well and the practitioner can achieve what he set out to do in perhaps thirty minutes; yet in other cases it may take an hour or more.

What happens during a treatment?

First of all, the pulses are read, and the practitioner will need to ask questions to ascertain how the patient is progressing after previous treatment. Needles will then be inserted or moxa applied until the desired effect has been achieved. Sometimes needles are only left in for a second or two, other times for a few minutes, and on occasions in excess of half an hour. The response to all the treatment is then assessed by reading the pulses again and by observing changes in the patient's colour, odour, sound and emotion. Meanwhile, the patient simply relaxes while the needles and moxa are doing their work.

Does the patient lie down or sit up for treatment?

This depends upon the patient. In the majority of cases the patient is encouraged to lie down so that he or she can be totally relaxed. But there are occasions when it is deemed necessary for the patient to be treated sitting up.

Are patients usually nervous about treatment?

Yes, I think most patients are nervous. In fact, I am sure that nine out of ten people think that insertion of the needle will be as painful as a hypodermic injection. We encourage our practitioners, after carrying out the initial examination consultation, to show the patient the needle and to demonstrate an insertion (although this is not done on a meridian or an acupuncture point since it may inappropriately influence the energy). Then the patient will come for the first treatment feeling more confident and relaxed. After that first experience, people are usually very happy about further treatments.

55

How quickly can a patient hope to feel improvement?

This again varies a good deal, speed of improvement depending on the type and severity of the disorder and on the state of the patient. Some patients feel changes right from the first treatment but usually one expects to feel benefit within four or five treatments.

The first benefits noticed are not necessarily improvements in the symptoms themselves. Often a patient feels better able to relax, has more vitality, feels more at peace, or feels more enjoyment in life. All these are positive signs that the *Ch'i* energy is being restored to balance; this will then naturally be followed by improvement in the symptoms.

Should the patient expect any adverse reaction to the treatment?

On the whole, any discomforts caused are mild and do not prevent the patient from continuing normal daily life. There can sometimes be an aggravation or a worsening of the symptoms; but this does not last long. The patient is usually told whether to expect such a reaction at the time of the treatment.

Any such aggravation can, in fact, be taken as an encouraging sign. It shows that the condition is responding to treatment and that it can be helped or cured. The aggravation can be seen as 'a healing crisis', evidence that the balance of energy is being restored.

As I say, any such aggravation usually brings only slight discomfort. But, it should be added that, in certain cases of deep-seated disease, reaction can be quite severe. It will, however, only last for a short time; perhaps from an hour to a day. Obviously, the practitioner tries to avoid causing such severe reaction but sometimes he has no choice. As someone who had been seriously ill for six years said to me once, 'The important question is, can you help me to get better? I certainly won't mind any temporary discomfort if I know that I am ultimately going to get well.'

Are there likely to be other effects besides these aggravations?

Yes, possibly. A patient may experience certain reactions to the adjusting balance of the energy, apart from possible aggravation of the symptoms. He or she may feel unusually tired and sleepy after the first treatments (and may be advised to go home and have a rest for an hour or so). Or treatment may cause looseness of the bowels, a cold, skin irritation or spots, or sweating. All of these effects are signs that the patient is responding to the treatment and is getting rid of toxic matter and poisons.

Such reactions depend largely on the disordered organ or function being treated. For example, a woman suffering a lot of pain and heavy bleeding during menstruation, and having the spleen or stomach treated to correct the disorder, might be surprised to find that she has a sudden desire for sweet things instead of the spicy foods which she has always previously preferred (or, *vice versa,* a sudden desire for spicy foods and no inclination for the sweet things that she has always been tempted to eat). Such reactions are only temporary and a natural balance will be reached as soon as the organ is functioning correctly.

It should be borne in mind that the practitioner's aim is gradually to balance the *whole* body, mind and spirit. All local reactions and aggravations resulting from treatment are caused by specific adjustments to the flow of energy in particular organs and functions. Finally, it should be emphasized that many people experience no aggravation or reaction.

THE LAW OF CURE

To understand the effects of treatment better, it would be helpful to mention here one of the important laws of traditional medicine. This states that if a cure is to be effected, then the disease must proceed from within outwards, from above to below, and that symptoms will return during treatment in reverse order from that in which they appeared. This is referred to as The Law of Cure.

This law is of practical importance during acupuncture

treatment. If you had an illness in the past – measles, for example – that your body dealt with naturally and overcame, then that illness will have been cleared from your system and will be no further problem to you. But if for any reason the illness was only suppressed and natural cure was blocked in some way, then, although the illness may have appeared to get better (that is, that the symptoms disappeared), the disease may in fact have been pushed deeper inside. Illnesses and diseases are frequently suppressed by drugs, for example. A fever may be forced down instead of reaching its natural crisis and is therefore not cleared from the body. Prevention of natural cure may also be caused by x-rays, radiotherapy, shock, innoculations, vaccinations, and so on.

As the acupuncture practitioner starts to treat a patient and the body begins to rebalance and heal itself, then a problem that was suppressed or blocked earlier in life may re-emerge. (It might help to visualize peeling an onion; as you start to peel, any disease that has been suppressed and held in a particular layer reappears as you reach that layer). Re-emergence of a suppressed problem – physical, mental or spiritual – is a good sign. It means that the body, mind and spirit are doing their best to heal, clearing old problems as they work themselves out from within.

Let us take a hypthetical case. Imagine that Mrs B. is seeking treatment for a chronic chest complaint; she has suffered from this complaint for the last seven or eight years. During the initial consultation we note that she had very bad eczema when she was in her teens and that this was successfully treated by the use of a cortisone-based cream. What really happened, however, was that, although the eczema was cleared from the skin by the cream, the *cause* of the eczema was ignored and not treated. As a result, it was suppressed and driven deeper into the body, mind and spirit. It is understandable, therefore, that, many years later, further symptoms should appear. But this time, they do not appear on the surface of the body, the skin, but deep inside, in the lungs. (The skin is regarded in traditional Chinese medicine as being an extension of the lungs). As Mrs B. is treated by acupuncture we expect the chest complaint to start improving; but, at some stage during the treatment, we would not be surprised if the eczema reappears. This is what is meant by the Law of Cure – that it comes from within outwards.

To take another situation – an arthritic condition may start improving in the shoulder, only to become simultaneously worse in the hands. This again would be a sign that the disease was being overcome – moving out of the body from above to below. A suppressed problem may manifest physically, but it may well have its mental or emotional counterpart. So, during treatment, a patient may experience recurrence of an emotional trauma not completely dealt with when it first occurred – an old fear, or an unresolved grief or an unforgiven anger, etcetera. These old, unresolved problems may return fleetingly during treatment, just for an hour or so, or maybe a little longer; it depends on how easily the patient's body, mind and spirit takes to deal with the problem. If, originally, the problem was severe and lasted for years, then it may take a fair amount of treatment by the practitioner and supportive work by the patient to clear it. The important factor is that the patient understands what is happening, knows what to expect. He or she can welcome the return of old problems, given satisfaction that all is moving in the right direction – towards cure.

There are just a few cases where, because of this process, the patient may not be advised to go ahead with acupuncture. If, for example, an elderly person is coping reasonably well with present symptoms with the help of drugs – with, say, asthma – then it may be foolish to disturb the energy and start this healing, clearing action – if there is a history of bad eczema and psoriasis. It may be felt that the person would be worse off if there were a return of these symptoms. With the younger person, however, in most cases it is well worth coping with the temporary discomfort of clearing the disease in depth because it provides sound investment for future health.

Can acupuncture do any harm, or cause harmful side effects?

I would refer here back to the chapter where I talked about symptomatic acupuncture. If traditional acupuncture is being practised then the patient will only have the type of reaction and aggravation described above. It is impossible for any harm to be done by the treatment. However, if 'local–doctor' or symptomatic acupuncture (not treating the cause) is practised, then treatment can be harmful, since it may worsen the underlying imbalance. Although such 'first–aid' treatment may bring temporary relief to the symptoms, it may do damage in the long term to the patient's energy balance and health. It is important, therefore, to make sure that the practitioner is fully qualified in the practice of traditional Chinese acupuncture – which seeks to remove the cause of the illness, not just to remove symptoms.

Is there the possibility of infection from the needles?

Tremendous emphasis is placed during training upon the need to sterilize needles (see p.40). Clinical hygiene is of paramount importance. Every properly-trained practitioner must comply with the code of practice laid down by his or her college and with the clinical requirements of local and national health authorities. Strict adherence to these codes of practice is also supervised by the Traditional Acupuncture Society, and the other two professional acupuncture societies (see p.97).

Should I stop taking drugs when I am having acupuncture treatment?

No, indeed not. It is dangerous to stop taking drugs without permission. (This is an extremely important subject and I discuss it fully in the next chapter.)

What about 'social drugs'? Can I continue to smoke and drink as usual?

The acupuncture practitioner will only make stipulation in such matters if he or she feels that they are genuinely interfering with treatment.

As I have said before, in the vast majority of cases, as

patients become more balanced in themselves, they find that the need or the desire to take 'social drugs' is considerably reduced. They either cut down the intake or give up such habits as a matter of course. Initially the practitioner will not be dogmatic about such habits unless the patient's health is in jeopardy or because the treatment is being hindered.

Does acupuncture do away with the need for medicines?

Not necessarily. It may occasionally be necessary to give some form of internal medicine along with the acupuncture treatment. This will be prescribed by the acupuncture practitioner and will be part of his whole plan for treating the patient. Such medicine will be of natural origin, such as prescribed in Western herbal medicine and homoeopathy.

Nevertheless, a large number of patients are already taking manufactured Western medication when they seek help from acupuncture. This should not be stopped abruptly but should be slowly reduced as the patient is able to function without its support. This is invariably done in cooperation with the patient's own general practitioner. It must be emphasized that it is dangerous to discontinue prescribed medication without consultation.

Is there an age limit for receiving treatment? Is acupuncture safe for children? Does it take longer for an older patient to get better?

There is no age limit, but a practitioner would not normally treat a child under seven years of age unless and until he or she has had considerable experience in practice. How long it takes to get better depends more on how long the patient has had the trouble than his or her age. A person of seventy with a disease of a year's duration should get well faster than a patient of thirty with a complant of ten years' duration. There is no definite guide that one can rely on with certainty; each person is a unique individual and each will respond differently irrespective of age, sex or anything else.

Are there any instructions or recommendations one should follow during a course of treatment?

Yes. These are some of the things to do and not to do:

It is better not to bathe on the day of treatment. A light shower is permissible (perhaps a couple of hours before or after).

Do not arrive rushed or hurried for treatment.

Do not eat a heavy meal before treatment or for an hour or two afterwards.

Do not give blood on the same day as having treatment.

After treatment, take things gently and quietly for an hour or two. (Following some treatments, specific guidelines, instructions or advice are given on an individual basis.)

Is there any way in which one can help a treatment to progress satisfactorily?

This question is answered fully in chapter 11 (Prevention of Disease), but, briefly, I must mention again the importance of moderation in habits, diet and lifestyle. It is difficult for any system of medicine to combat the effects of the stresses generated by the way of life that many people adopt today. Whilst it is unfair to expect people to change their lifestyles dramatically overnight, we can at least be aware that these stresses do have their effect and can try not to allow them to dominate our lives.

Our *Ch'i* energy is replenished by the food we eat and the air we breathe. And, if the organs or the 'officials' (regulators) of the body, mind and spirit are to do their work well, they must be refuelled with vital *Ch'i* energy of high quality. You would not expect a Rolls Royce to run well on two-star petrol or paraffin, and we should not expect body, mind and spirit to function on an impure diet and stale air. We need good quality nourishment of all kinds – for mental and spiritual as well as physical well-being. And plenty of fresh air and exercise.

In general, we need to aim for a balanced diet. Try to replace some of the highly-processed foods with more natural forms of the same food. Replace white flour and sugar with whole-meal flour and brown sugar. Avoid eating too many 'convenience' foods, such as those which have been pre-cooked, packaged, frozen or tinned. Do not overcook vegetables as this destroys a lot of their valuable nutrients. But do not become a slave to food and go to extremes of food 'faddism'; this can do more harm than good.

It helps just to look at what it is we are eating. We can be quite shocked when we realise the sum total of garbage we are consuming. With just a little effort, some of this rubbish can be replaced by more nutritious food – food which is just as enjoyable.

9   The Taking of Drugs while having Acupuncture Treatment

I have seen leaflets which advocate dispensing with all drugs when having acupuncture treatment. Is this the correct thing to do?

As I said in the last chapter, no, it is not the correct thing to do. I regard any such statement as being both irresponsible and dangerous. A large number of patients who come for traditional Chinese acupuncture are taking some form of medically-prescribed drug and we must recognise that many of them are only able to survive because of that drug. The dosage of these drugs varies greatly, as does the type of drug, and it is important that the patient should tell his or her acupuncture practitioner exactly what drugs or medicines are being taken and in what dosage.

Broadly speaking, we see these drugs as falling into two categories. First there are those prescribed for ease of pain, tension and stress, etcetera; second, there are the life-support drugs, such as insulin, steroids, and so on. It will be easy and safe for the patient to withdraw slowly from the former group of drugs as he or she will find that the need for them decreases according to response to treatment. But premature withdrawal from the second category of drug could seriously endanger the health or even the life of the patient. As acupuncture treatment progresses, it may well prove possible to decrease the amounts of these drugs being taken; but this must be done exceedingly carefully, and slowly, and the effects must be thoroughly monitored throughout.

An acupuncturist will certainly not recommend any reduction until he finds that the patient is responding to treatment and that the organ or function which was requiring help from the drugs is getting stronger. At this point, he would hope to try a small reduction of the drugs. Wherever possible, this reduction is done with the cooperation and approval of the doctor or specialist who prescribed the drugs in the first place.

On no account should any patient, in a mood of enthusiastic optimism, suddenly stop taking his or her drugs. To do so can place a big strain on the body, and it will certainly hinder rather than help recovery by creating some form of crisis.

It is important to make clear that being a practitioner of natural healing does not mean being anti-drugs. This would be an exceedingly foolish stance. Even if not in the life-support category, drugs can be exceedingly helpful, especially for acute conditions. For example, a sleeping tablet taken after a time of particular stress and hardship may be an excellent means for giving the body, the mind and the spirit a chance to rest and recover from a temporary and transient blow. It would not, however, be sensible medical practice to give a person sleeping tablets for five years because he is unable to sleep (as, unfortunately, has been the experience of many of my patients). It would be better practice to find the cause of the inability to sleep and to try to remedy that.

Is it all right to take the occasional aspirin or indigestion tablet while undergoing acupuncture treatment?

During the time you are undergoing acupuncture treatment, it is really best for you to consult with your practitioner before taking any form of medication. You will ideally have told the acupuncturist of any drugs that you have been taking, as prescribed by your doctor, and the practitioner will have planned his treatment taking this into account. But if you then add any new drug on your own initiative, without his knowledge, this can confuse the picture and possibly interfere with the progress of the treatment.

Perhaps the most important aspect of this discipline is that the patient may be having some form of temporary treatment reaction or aggravation, or may be having some form of Law of Cure response. Thus, if the patient does not realise that the catarrh, or the headache, or the skin rash, or the diarrhoea is a direct result of the treatment, he or she may decide to dose himself (or even go to his doctor for a prescription). To take drugs at this point would only suppress the symptoms and push the disease back inside again, just as the body was beginning to deal with it, work it out and overcome it naturally. For healing to take place, it is important to allow any such reaction to take its natural course.

But, if in doubt, consult your practitioner. For care should be taken also not to err in the other direction – to assume that every ill that befalls you during the time you are undergoing acupuncture treatment *is* the result of the treatment. You could genuinely have caught a cold, or the 'flu, or have a hangover, developed shingles, have food poisoning, or whatever. Medication may well be needed in this new circumstance, so keep your practitioner informed – because he will then be able to treat these developments if they arise – on top of the original cause for which he is essentially treating you.

10 Different Ways in which Acupuncture can be Used

You mentioned earlier that some acupuncturists treat the symptoms of illness rather than concerning themselves with the cause of it. Could you say a little more about this?

It is extremely important to make clear that acupuncture can be used in two distinct and totally different ways. And there are certain dangers in using acupuncture in one of these ways – that is, when it is used with the sole aim of removing symptoms.

I need to come back briefly to consideration of disease and its cause. As I have explained, if the energy in a meridian becomes imbalanced then, after a time, the person will start noticing signs of distress. Quite simply, this is the body or the mind or the spirit saying something is going wrong, please help. Now the sign may be a physical one or it may be an emotional or a mental one; but all of them are the first symptoms of disease. They are warning or distress signals.

If nothing is done to help, then the situation worsens and finally a recognisable pattern of symptoms develops – which may be labelled rheumatoid arthritis, lumbago, migraine, or any one of the countless, named diseases.

It is obvious that if the person is going to get better the cause of illness must be dealt with and if possible removed. Then, when the energy is rebalanced by acupuncture, the symptoms will disappear, the person will get better, and stay better.

This was the aim of the Chinese when they first used acupuncture. The practice of traditional Chinese acupuncture deals with the whole person and the object is to discover the underlying cause of disease and to deal directly with that cause.

Thus, the first concern is not treating to relieve symptoms if, in so doing, the disease is in fact suppressed.

Traditional acupuncture, instead of asking 'What kind of symptoms does this person have?' asks 'What kind of person has these symptoms, and why?'

It takes a long time to train practitioners properly in this system of medicine. The Chinese themselves believe it takes twenty years to become really proficient. Although the theory of traditional acupuncture is relatively simple, practice of it is complex. For example, it is not easy to learn how to read the pulses and the state of the energy, to ascertain the primary energy imbalance and to work out the necessary treatment. It is not easy to learn to analyse the sounds, colours, emotions and odours. That is why it takes so long to become a master of acupuncture.

I am stating this because I feel it is part of the reason why another type of acupuncture – 'formula acupuncture' – is frequently practised in the West. People have seen fine results from acupuncture practised by a traditional practitioner and, in their wish to help people in a similar way, they have tried to watch, remember and copy the masters' treatments. But, in fact, one can gain very little real understanding simply from observing other practitioners and their treatments because in traditional acupuncture no two people are ever treated in the same way. Each person is unique, and will require individual treatment. It can be quite inappropriate therefore to use formula treatments for common symptoms.

Nevertheless, the Chinese have, over the centuries, collected and approved numerous formulae for specific problems. However, the traditionally-trained Chinese acupuncturist knows so much about the concepts and practice of acupuncture that he is able to diagnose accurately first on traditional principles and then select the appropriate formula. In the West, these formulae are being used quite inappropriately. There are many people practising acupuncture who have done as little as a weekend or just one week's training; or perhaps they have visited China for a few weeks. They feel that they are competent acupuncturists but, in fact, their practice is simply based on remembering and using formulae for symptoms and labelled diseases. Such a practitioner simply looks up, say, 'migraine' in his little book and then tries any formula list of points suggested as being helpful.

Not only is this foolish but, as I have said before, it can, in many cases, be harmful. Simply to use a list of points for relieving migraine on all patients suffering from that symptom is to deny the individuality of each one. No two migraines derive from exactly the same causes. One person's migraine may be caused by an overload of worry, another's may be caused by too much rich, fatty food, and another's may be caused through taking drugs. The trouble may perhaps be in the spleen, or it may be in the liver, or it may be in the gall bladder, or it may be in the bladder, or it may be in the small intestines. How can two people with the symptom 'migraine' possibly be cured by using the same points?

If an inadequately trained practitioner does treat on the basis of the symptom, and selects a generally-applicable formula supposedly helpful for this symptom, then it is possible, even likely, that the patient's energy will become further imbalanced rather than balanced. Even if the symptom disappears, it is quite possible that in a few months' or a year's time further problems will develop that may be of an even more serious nature (owing to the worsened imbalance of energy caused by the symptomatic acupuncture).

In the Far East, as I have said, traditional acupuncture does acknowledge and permit 'local-doctor' or formula acupuncture, but only as a temporary or 'first aid' measure. Suppose you have a headache – perhaps due to staying up too late, or drinking a little bit too much, or because of shock or unusual stress; you might take an aspirin or a Disprin, which would then remove the headache. In such a case, Far Eastern practice might well be to use a formula treatment just to remove the headache, an equivalent to the Disprin. But if you have repetitive headaches then you would certainly not continue just taking Disprin; you would seek help from your family physician. Likewise, in the Far East, the sufferer of continual headaches would seek the help of the traditional medical practitioner.

I will tell you of an actual case which demonstrates the

two types of acupuncture. A thirty-eight year old American doctor from New York took a very brief course in acupuncture; I think it lasted about ten days. She learned where the acupuncture points are located and was given a list of points that would help specific problems. She herself had had a recurrent knee problem over the previous five years and decided to treat herself with acupuncture. Over a period of several weeks, she stimulated several points located around the knee and her pain and problem seemed to clear completely. About a year later she had a heart attack. The cause was a mystery to the specialists. There were apparently no factors in her life, her present state of health, or her family history that could account for her having any heart problem. It was simply inexplicable. But no one had considered the fact that she had given herself acupuncture. It is most likely that her heart attack was caused, or contributed to, by this symptomatic acupuncture. Heavy local stimulation of these points every day could easily have given rise to a serious imbalance of the heart energy and thus put the heart itself under considerable stress.

When energy is directed to one part of the body to relieve pain, it has to be borne in mind that that energy must come from another part of the body. In the above case, it may well have been that the heart meridian was being directly robbed of its energy.

So, you see that this wonderful system of medicine can easily be misused and abused. The practice of it in the West is further complicated by the fact that we have a different view of, and attitude to, health and disease from the Chinese. For us, the quickest possible alleviation of symptoms is often the only health care that we afford ourselves. The Western and Eastern medical systems tend to tackle ill health from opposite viewpoints. The Western doctor is trained to treat particular disorders. Thus we have cardiac specialists, renal specialists, ophthalmologists, neurologists, and so on, each with special knowledge and skills at his disposal. The physician prescribes drugs to kill infection, to ease pain, to check symptoms and he caters for deficiencies (e.g. hormone deficiency). The surgeon operates to remove diseased parts of the body and to repair parts which have broken down, and so on.

But, as I have said, the traditional Chinese doctor looks

upon symptoms only as an *indication* of trouble, not as being in themselves the trouble. He is trained to seek that which is causing the symptom, and his treatment aims to deal primarily with that cause and only secondarily with the symptoms.

Because of this fundamentally different approach to illness and disease, it is exceedingly difficult for a Western-trained doctor to learn, properly understand and practise traditional acupuncture. Symptomatic acupuncture on the other hand, slips much more easily into his present system of medicine. To the Western-trained doctor it seems perfectly reasonable that there is a particular formula treatment for migraine, another for lumbago, another for arthritis, and so on. He is happy therefore to learn how to find the acupuncture points and to use them in this way.

At present, there is growing interest in acupuncture in the West. In the medical profession, many doctors are wanting to add acupuncture to their skills and to make it available in hospitals. Unfortunately, more and more of them are doing short training courses and are generally practising symptomatic acupuncture only. They are ignorant of the dangers of this method and ignorant of the way in which traditional acupuncture should be practised.

A further point is that it is simply not sensible for any person to try to practise both Eastern and Western medicine at the same time. Very few Western doctors, having spent seven to ten years in training, are willing to spend the necessary further five to ten years studying traditional acupuncture properly (unless they are dissatisfied with the Western system, and wish to change over completely). Apart from that, Western medicine is of little or no help in practising acupuncture. As I have described, the concepts are totally different.

In China, all medical students have the same basic training in anatomy, physiology, pathology and other subjects. They then specialize in *either* Western medicine *or* traditional Chinese medicine. When qualified, they practise side by side, and they decide together whether traditional medicine or modern medicine offers the better prospect for a particular patient. But neither attempts to learn or practise both.

If this principle does not become understood and practised

in the West, it will mean that very poor acupuncture will be administered by many Western doctors in their practices and in the hospitals of this country. Unfortunately, acupuncture will then be widely judged on that unsatisfactory basis. It will be natural, too, for people to assume that any acupuncture treatment given by their doctors will automatically be good and completely safe. As I have explained, this may well not be the case. It can only be good acupuncture if the practitioner involved has had an absolute minimum of three years' training at a recognized college and is not practising symptomatic or formula treatment.

We can imagine that originally, in ancient China, there were people who, without special study, picked up a little knowledge about acupuncture. They noticed that a particular treatment was effective for relieving earache, another helped colic, another helped headache, and so on. So there grew up the practice of treating one's family, or of someone taking on responsibility for treating minor ailments in the local community. Anyone practising in this way was known as a local doctor, or barefoot doctor. The need for such a system in China's vast rural communities becomes apparent when we realize that the nearest qualified practitioner was quite likely to have been hundreds of miles away. Local doctor treatment was therefore regarded as an important emergency or first-aid service, effective until such time as a fully qualified traditional acupuncturist could be reached if required.

There is still a need for this type of acupuncture in China today since its vast rural populations cannot possibly be catered for in any other way. But this is not appropriate or necessary in the West. Western doctors giving symptomatic treatment for serious ailments after inadequate training is akin to a first-aid man attempting surgery. Good, effective and safe acupuncture, giving long-term benefit, requires thorough traditional training.

There has been a lot of publicity lately about ear staples to help you to lose weight, or to give up smoking or alcohol. What do you think about this?

To put a staple in an acupuncture point of the ear in order to stop a person from eating, or drinking alcohol, or smoking, is again an endeavour to treat symptoms. It is simply another example of symptomatic acupuncture.

We have to ask ourselves why the person is drinking alcohol or smoking excessively, or is over-indulging in food? Usually, all these habits are crutches to help people to keep going. No person in a reasonable state of body, mind or spirit needs to indulge in alcohol to an extent where it is likely to make him a burden on his family, himself and the community.

We use the statement that people are 'driven to drink'; and in many cases this is certainly true. A person may suffer such pain in mind, or body or spirit that he needs an escape from it. He feels he needs the support of alcohol in order to function and to deal with the anguish. The same applies with food. So many desperately sick people seek comfort in food – to fill the void, to alleviate the sense of emptiness. The food becomes a crutch or a dummy. Similar reasons underlie the compulsion to smoke excessively.

I know of people who have had symptomatic treatment in order to lose weight, or to stop smoking or drinking. The treatment was in some cases effective; but it took away the crutch only, which in turn resulted in severe mental breakdown.

Such reactions emphasize the importance of seeking to have the *cause* of the excessive habit treated. Remove the cause and then the desire to smoke, or drink, or eat excessively will disappear. Remove the symptoms by suppressing the desire and it will surely break out in some other way.

One of the practices first filmed and written about by Western people who have visited Red China in recent years has been the use of acupuncture for anaesthesia. Is this a part of the work of the traditional acupuncturist?

This is a different and particular use of acupuncture. Strictly

73

speaking, this practice should be called acupuncture analgesia, because the patient is not anaesthetized. The patient is conscious during the operation and merely loses sensation of pain in a specific part of the body. It has been much talked about in the West because the techniques are relatively new and have been much publicised by China.

Acupuncturists in modern China have been researching old methods and have been experimenting to find ways to anaesthetize different parts of the body needing surgery. It is done quite simply – by placing acupuncture needles into specific points of the body. Very often only two, or perhaps four, needles are inserted, usually in the lower legs and the feet, or the lower arms, or the ears. These needles are then stimulated, each in turn, for some fifteen to twenty minutes before the operation (and then at intervals during the operation). The stimulation can either be carried out by hand or by using a machine.

The practice is proving very successful. The patients are conscious during the operation and appear to be completely calm and relaxed about it. Blood pressure, breathing and pulse remain normal. In many cases the patient actively cooperates with the surgeon (in regulating his own breathing, for instance).

There is still sensation in the anaesthetized area, but no pain is felt. When an incision is made by the surgeon, it feels to the patient as though a pencil is being run across the skin. He can be aware that an organ is being moved, or that bone is being cut, but that is all. In China, this method of anaesthesia is proving particularly valuable in isolated rural areas where it is either impossible to get patients needing urgent operations to a hospital or there is not time to get other anaesthesia equipment to the location. A large number of lives have been saved through using this technique.

In the West, acupuncture analgesia should also have a part to play. It would make it possible to operate on patients whose age, heart condition, and so on, would expose them to serious danger if conventional anaesthetics were used. Such people are at present condemned to lives of misery because there is no alternative form of anaesthesia available.

Acupuncture analgesia has several other advantages. It is not

Acupuncture analgesia has several other advantages. It is not only much less expensive than conventional methods but it has the great merit that the patient suffers no side- or after-effects from it. In an emergency, an operation can be performed immediately as there are none of the usual empty-stomach requirements. A patient may eat at any time before or after an operation. Recovery time after minor operations is very much reduced. Patients frequently feel well enough to walk from the operating table back to their hospital beds.

Nevertheless, I would like to mention a possible reservation about its use in the West. Maybe because we are conditioned to be afraid of pain, and because we hear about, think about and perhaps see the traumas associated with major surgery, it may be too much to expect us to accept the prospect of being conscious during surgery (especially since the analgesic effect can sometimes suddenly wear off during the operation).

Acupuncture analgesia can be used very successfully during childbirth. The mother can be fully conscious, during the delivery, of all that is happening, and yet can be free of any pain. There is the added advantage that drugs will not then be needed. Acupuncture for childbirth could easily become a major contribution to Western health care as people can be trained in the use of it in a fairly short time. It is not necessary to undertake the full training required to become a traditional acupuncturist. Such a practitioner would be using acupuncture for this one purpose only, and would not be concerned with diagnosis and treatment of illness.

So acupuncture analgesia is really a practice quite distinct from traditional acupuncture, or even 'local-doctor', or barefoot acupuncture. If a person has received acupuncture analgesia for surgery, dental work, or childbirth, he or she should be checked over later by a practising acupuncturist to make sure that the energy has rebalanced itself after the analgesia. (Only occasionally is a balancing treatment needed). This check should be seen as a safeguard for the person's future welfare.

11 The Prevention of Disease

If a person has acupuncture treatment early enough, can disease be prevented from developing?

In many cases, certainly. Prevention is really the root concept and main purpose underlying traditional Chinese acupuncture. It should ideally be seen and primarily used as a preventative medicine.

The practitioner will be able to tell from the pulses and by other diagnostic means if any aspect of the person is not in correct working order long before disease seriously develops. I described earlier how the Chinese found that, if the twelve organs and functions are working together in balance and harmony, then it is impossible for there to be illness in the body, the mind, or the spirit. Every single disease known to mankind results from one or more of these organs and functions having energy imbalance. Thus, if the practitioner can detect the first signs of imbalance, he will be able to correct it and give the body a chance to return to normal functioning, thus preventing disease from developing.

It sounds as though regular check-ups would be valuable. Is an acupuncture practitioner willing to give a person just a check-up from time to time, to find out if there is anything starting to go wrong?

Yes, indeed. He or she would be only too happy to do so. The great strength, joy and assurance of traditional acupuncture is that it is a system of health care and disease prevention. The

76

ancient Chinese visited their acupuncturists at the change of each season (see ch. 3) so that the practitioner could check for any signs of imbalance and correct it. This is still the practice in modern China.

When you think about it, we care for our cars by regularly taking them along to a garage for servicing so that they can continue to give us good performance. If the mechanic advises work should be done on the car, we do not hesitate to let him go ahead. But what do we do about our most precious possessions – our body, mind and spirit? What do we do with them? Do we keep a watchful eye on them and take them along for a servicing, so that they can continue to enjoy long years of happy, healthy life? You have only to go and look into a doctor's surgery to see the number of people who have waited until too late, until the damage has developed and the body's mechanism has broken down. Only then have they paid attention. (Not that they can be held entirely to blame. Western medicine continually places more emphasis on, and devotes more resources to, the cure of disease rather than the maintenance of health).

The Chinese have been much wiser. It was because of the acupuncturist's ability to prevent illness that people used to visit and pay him only when they were well. Indeed, it is said that if they became ill, then the practitioner's services were dispensed with. (In the case of the mandarin classes, sometimes the practitioner himself was dispensed with!) But implicit in this view of the doctor's responsibility was the understanding that it is not enough just to have a periodic check-up and treatment to avoid illness; people knew that they had to play *their* part – to follow the guidance of the doctor, to be constantly alert to the functioning of body, mind and spirit, and to their inter-relationship with others and the environment.

You said at the beginning of the book that the acupuncturist must understand why a person's energy has become imbalanced. Presumably the person should also understand the cause of the imbalance if he or she is not to slip back again into the same imbalance?

That is right. It is only too easy for the person to become

imbalanced again unless he has understood why it came about in the first place and has taken steps to prevent its recurrence. If we are to prevent disease we need to understand the cause ourselves. We need to ask ourselves, 'How did this illness come about?'

So what is it that upsets the functioning of the twelve meridians or pathways of energy and causes them to become imbalanced?

There are two aspects in answer to this.

The first is the way a person lives his life. This is the more general aspect. The Chinese see that the energy flowing through the twelve meridians is susceptible to stress, strain and trauma. All ill health is seen as attributable to these factors. (That is, of course, apart from illness caused by mechanical or chemical injury).

The second aspect we must consider is that the person may be suffering from a disease in body, mind, or spirit. Disease, the Chinese believe, is caused by interaction between the internal condition of a person and the external world; and there are certain internal and external factors (seven of each) which may bring it about. Internally, for example, balance of energy can be affected by an excess of fear, grief, anger, joy, worry or anxiety; and it may be affected by hereditary constitutional factors. Externally, it may be affected by environmental changes; these, traditionally, were categorized as cold, heat, dryness, humidity, damp, wind and fire.

At certain times, we are all exposed to every one of these internal and external factors, and a healthy body, mind and spirit will be able to cope with them. For example, we sometimes become worried, or we become exposed to excessive heat or damp; but, after a short time, our minds and bodies adjust and we do not suffer ill-effect from the experience. But, when body, mind, or spirit is subjected to continual excess of any internal or external factor, then this can cause serious imbalance of the *Ch'i* energy, and disease symptoms will appear in the body, the mind or the spirit.

In the case of infectious and contagious disease, the Chinese believe that, if a person is in as near perfect health as possible, the body will be able to resist disease. It is the fact that resistance has been lowered by one of the above factors that allows the disease to take hold. To stay healthy we need to be able to move and change with the circumstances, and not become overwhelmed by stressful factors to the point where we lose resilience and cannot recover normal energy balance.

So what can be done to avoid imbalance? What did the Chinese do themselves?

The Chinese understood that they were part of everything and were affected by everything. They did not see themselves as we often do today – so individually separate and isolated. They also saw that they had a responsibility for their own health; very different again from us today, where we place responsibility for our health on the doctor. It was very important to the Chinese to know how to keep well and balanced.

Consider first their pace of living. This was, of course, much slower than ours. People grew up believing that order, tranquillity, happiness (and consequently health) stemmed from the effort of each individual to follow the *Tao* (see chapter 13). Each person's primary intent was to bring about and keep balance and harmony within himself, and within his life. Ideally, such balance and harmony would then spread out in ever-widening circles – out into the family and the home, out into the communities of village and town, and on and on through the whole country. It would uphold and influence all aspects of work, all the needs of family and neighbours, all the policies in government of the country. And it would influence production of all the necessities of life and works of art. This philosophy meant living in accord with Nature, and being obedient to natural laws.

Life is always moving and flowing, from day to night, from activity to rest, from joy to sadness, from *yang* to *yin*. Thus everything passes. The Chinese saw that it was pointless to become too attached to success and ambition, for tomorrow there could be failure. It was foolish to boast of having something, for tomorrow it could be gone. Thus they accepted the natural law, the coming and the passing, whether good or bad.

In order to follow the *Tao,* therefore, the ancient Chinese emphasized the need for moderation in all things; an avoidance of all excesses. They generally sought to live and eat simply; very rarely would they overtax their minds or their bodies; and certainly they would not do so striving for excessive gains.

Through their understanding of the natural laws and the seven internal and external causative factors of disease (p.78), they were able to understand any signs of disease in themselves. They took heed of any small symptoms – such as a headache, going off their food, an abnormal temperature, or whatever; and if possible they dealt with them themselves. They considered what was going on in their lives, what they had eaten, the season, the time of day, the weather. And they tried to counter the causes of their symptoms by obeying Nature's message. The symptoms could have been due to too much stress or over-work; or to too much food or the wrong kind of food. Some foods are helpful for feverish conditions; some for cold and numb conditions, and aching limbs. Some are helpful for cleansing or for building up the blood. Some strengthen and give energy, and some quieten the energy down. So they would consider their diet, their food, their exercise, their behaviour, their breathing, their bowels, and so on, to see if they could determine the reason for the illness.

The Chinese also observed that the development of disease is slow. There may be signs of disorder months or even years before serious disease is recognized. Any recurring symptom, however small, should be taken as a valuable warning sign, as a distress signal from the body or mind or spirit saying that all is not well within. Then there is usually plenty of time to discover the hidden cause of the problem, before the early symptoms give way to the more serious illness of which they are a warning.

It was only when people were not able to sort things out for themselves that they sought the help of the doctor of traditional Chinese medicine. Through his skill and expertise, he was able to pinpoint the cause and set about correcting it.

Apart from acupuncture, his treatments included the use of herbs and the giving of massage, of dietary and physical exercise regimes, of breathing exercises, of medicine for better functioning of the bowels, and so on.

How can we make use of this knowledge here in the West to help prevent disease?

Once we understand that illness of the body, mind and spirit does not just happen – that it does not just come along from outside and attack us as if we have no responsibility for it – then we can be less afraid of it. We will then perhaps begin to take a little more responsibility for ourselves. We are generally inclined to think that colds, or headaches, or the irregularity of periods, or feelings of nausea, or fevers are things which just unfortunately happen. Even with more serious problems – like bronchitis, emphysema, even heart failure, arthritis or cancer – we still tend to feel they have nothing to do with any fault on our part. But such diseases are often the result of violent disregard for natural laws and a natural way of life. We do not usually see the connection between our way of life and our state of health. We need to make use of this knowledge as the ancient Chinese did.

We are inclined also to expect the doctor to make us well. We rely on him to step in and make us better. We hand over the burden of the responsibility to him (and may even blame him if he fails). We hope for some mysterious external power to cure us and leave it at that. How much better it would be if we were willing to work *with* the doctor, sought his guidance on how to keep well and accepted some of the responsibility for preventing our illnesses.

The attitude of expecting our health and well being to be looked after by someone else puts us outside of ourselves. Foregoing our own powers of self-help makes us unnecessarily afraid and helpless. The beauty of traditional Chinese acupuncture is that it does the opposite. It encourages us to look at ourselves and not to hide away; to help ourselves and to take responsibility for ourselves.

If we watch, we can see that we *are* affected by our circumstances, by our environment, and by other factors, both internal and external. There are times when we are aware that we are becoming unwell and it is then that we should take stock and endeavour to put right those factors which are causing the situation. Illness is not a mystery at all. It is simply a natural and lawful consequence of overloading body, mind and spirit. The message from the Chinese is to lead a life of moderation, and to live in harmony with the natural rhythms. To make this a little clearer, we need to consider what is meant by natural rhythms and moderation.

First, we need to consider the workings of *yin* and *yang* and the five elements. (I spoke of these in chapter 3). We can see the natural rhythm of *yin* and *yang* expressed in the alternation of day and night, and of activity and resting. And we see the natural rhythms of the five elements in the cycle of the seasons. But just imagine what it would be like if these natural rhythms were violated. Supposing the day continued right through the night, or that the night continued right through the day. Or supposing spring came again in place of autumn. There would be total chaos. Yet that is what we try to do. We are always trying to extend the day into the night, and the night into the day – being active when it is time to rest, and *vice versa*.

Just watch the children when they are tired. They just curl up and go to sleep. And when they are hungry, they eat; and as soon as they have had enough, they stop. This is obeying the natural rhythms of *yin* and *yang*. Yet we adults ignore this rhythm and moderation. We push ourselves to work when we are very tired. We stay up late into the night. Then we fall asleep when we should be up and about. We continue to eat when we are full, or we eat when we are not even hungry or fail to eat properly when we are hungry. We could make a never-ending list of all of such habits. We ignore Nature to do what we like; and we think we can reap a good harvest all the year round without fail, despite continual violation of natural laws.

And then consider what we do with our emotions. When a child is happy he laughs; when he is sad and hurt, he cries. But adults think it is not acceptable to be spontaneously natural.

We suppress tears, grief and anger, and we love spontaneously far too little. Thus we block the natural response and flow of the five elements.

Consider again the law of Midday and Midnight (p.27). If we were to pay a little more heed to our own natural clock, it would give us a guide to the right time (and the wrong time) to do things. It is following the natural rhythm and flow, and is to our advantage, if we eat well at the optimum time for the stomach; for example, between seven and nine o'clock in the morning. In other words, it is important to eat a good breakfast. It is better for us to evacuate the bowels between five and seven o'clock in the morning. It is easier for us to be sociable and alive between seven and eleven o'clock in the evening. And it is good for us to be in bed and asleep by eleven o'clock (so that the officials or regulators of the Wood element can deal with planning and decision-making when we are not too mentally or physically active. Too much activity at this time can give rise to insomnia).

Considering the seven internal and seven external causative factors of disease (p.78), we need to pay heed to balance and whether any factor is excessive. Have I been grieving for too long? Am I excessively worried and angry? Why am I so bothered by a damp house? Why do I always seem too cold?

And we must consider our lifestyle and our life situation, and how they may be affecting our health. What excessive strains and stresses am I being subjected to? Am I in a job that I resent and dislike? Am I having to cope with too much anger, resentment, hatred, envy, loneliness or grief? Am I working in bad conditions? Am I working excessively or am I not working hard enough? Do I have to cope with too many decisions, too much responsibility? Perhaps I am bored? Perhaps I am suffering from the competitive spirit of this day and age, struggling for qualifications, for recognition, for achievement, for power, for status?

So we need to remember the five elements. We can notice if any of our emotions are excessive or inappropriate. Am I always irritable? Am I always crying? Am I always complaining? Do I crave certain foods and certain flavours? Do I often feel too hot, or too cold? Any such signals should make us suspicious that there is imbalance, and that we should be willing to make changes to bring about better balance and harmony, and thus prevent illness.

At the present time, it is not easy to lead a naturally healthy life. The ideal would be for us to be eating much purer food, to be drinking purer water, breathing purer air, to be working at a pace and extent more in harmony with natural laws, free from excessive stress. We should be able to live in more tranquillity and happiness, closer to nature, creation and God.

Some of these things are not in our control and, of course, some difficulty, stress and anxiety cannot be avoided. Things do go wrong and accidents will happen; but we still can do a lot to improve our individual situations.

Perhaps the most important thing of all is to get values straight. Those people who have become dissatisfied with the technological rat-race and are seeking to find a richness and purpose in life in other ways, have already taken steps towards healthy living. *Where* they find quality in life is of little importance. They may find it in religion or philosophy, in art or music, or in a style of living closer to nature and natural laws. They may find it in the simple tasks of daily life, and in simple pleasures. Finding it somewhere is what matters.

Once this revaluation has happened, everything else falls into place. Our attitudes towards life, work, pleasure and possessions naturally alter. We cease to place such importance on pleasures and possessions. As we cease to work for what we can get out of life, we begin to discover the enjoyment of seeing what we can put into it. We find time again to enjoy the natural things that are freely given to all people – the sky, the birds, the trees, and above all the companionship of our fellow humans. We see more, hear more, and give more attention to what needs to be done. We begin to find a richness in life that eluded us when we were caught up in the rush and the bustle.

If we endeavour to change our values and outlook in such ways, we are moving towards a mental and spiritual harmony which automatically affects the state of the physical body. Our *Ch'i* energy becomes stronger and better balanced, thus enabling us to function at a much healthier level. Thus, reassessment of values is, in itself, a helpful step in taking care of body, mind and spirit.

To sum up, we can learn to take responsibility for our own health. We can look carefully at our own lifestyle and its stresses, and take notice of any symptoms of distress. We can also try to live in harmony with the natural cycles and laws of nature, letting them guide us to leading a moderate and a balanced way of life.

We can take better care of ourselves – our bodies, our minds, and our spirits – by allocating the appropriate time to work and to play, to exercise and to rest. This resting means sleeping in harmony with the cycles of earth and sun, and not trying to turn night into day or *vice versa*. And we can take time each day to be alone, and to be quiet, in order to refresh ourselves and become one with ourselves again.

DIET AND EATING HABITS

A further responsibility is the need to give attention to diet, and to eating habits. As I already have said, certain flavours correlate with certain elements. Thus it is helpful to eat a diet well-balanced from the point of view of flavour as well as nutrition. We should watch that we do not eat too many sweet foods, too many sour or bitter foods, too many hot and pungent foods, or take too much salt. All flavours in moderation.

The Chinese did, and still do, place enormous importance on the freshness of food. They try to eat their vegetables within a few hours of picking, and their meat within a few hours of killing. This is in order that they may be eating the food while the *Ch'i* energy is still vital within it. (They have vegetable markets twice a day for this reason). There is great wisdom in this practice, and we should make every effort to do the same. We must not depend so much on eating frozen, tinned, preserved foods; we must try to eat foods when they are fresh, which means buying particular foods during their appropriate season.

We can do our best to eat at regular times, and – above all – in moderation. We should remember that the stomach is best prepared for digesting food in the morning; much less so late in the evening. The common habit of eating a main meal in the evening is certainly not ideal from the health point of view. There is a wise saying, 'Eat breakfast like a king, lunch like a prince and supper like a pauper.' There is much sense in this.

In addition to ensuring that our diet is as wholesome and balanced as possible – and consists, as far as possible, of fresh foods – we also need to look for food which is uncontaminated by sprays, for food which does not contain too much chemical flavouring and colouring, and for food which is free of the preservatives and additives so often put into it for the sake of commercial convenience.

We should eat plenty of compost-grown whole cereals and grains from which nutrients, such as wheatgerm, have not been removed. Wholemeal bread and wholemeal flour products, unpolished rice, whole wheat, barley and rye, crushed oats – all these contribute immensely to a healthy diet. Legumes and certain seeds – such as split peas, beans, soya beans, lentils, nuts, sesame and sunflower seeds, Chinese sprouting beans – are very nutritious and are a valuable source of protein. If we supplement our diet with them, it becomes unnecessary to eat so much meat and cheese, both of which, if eaten in excess, put too much animal fat into the body. Plenty of vegetables should be the order of the day, along with salad and fruit (again, preferably fresh and in season). And, if we need to sweeten food, we should use pure brown sugar or honey.

In the West we are inclined to eat too much sweet and rich food. It is important that we do not overload our bodies with sugar, cakes, puddings, sweets, soft drinks and biscuits. Nor should we take in too much rich, fatty food – through consuming large quantities of butter, cream, rich milk, cheese, chocolate, or through cooking, especially frying, with butter, dripping and lard.

The final point on eating habits is that we should 'drink our food and eat our drinks.' This is a very old saying, but very wise. It means to say that we should chew food thoroughly, until it becomes liquid in the mouth; and that we should drink liquid slowly, a little at a time, holding it in the mouth long enough for it to become well mixed with saliva. The way we eat is perhaps as important as what we eat. The process of digestion and assimilation should be started correctly; this will not be so unless all food and liquid is adequately mixed with saliva in the mouth.

ELIMINATION

After considering diet and eating habits, we must give attention to elimination. Its importance cannot be stressed too strongly. The bowels, the bladder and the kidneys must be functioning properly. If there is any problem with them, one should take heed, and get advice and treatment. As stated earlier, when talking about the Chinese clock (p.26), a good time for movement of the bowels is between five o'clock and seven o'clock in the morning. I suggest that if you were to make a regular habit of eliminating during this period, giving yourself plenty of time, many of the problems of, and resulting from constipation, etcetera, would disappear. Elimination through the skin is also very important; the exreted wastes of sweating must be regularly washed away.

Failure to evacuate and eliminate waste products of the body can only mean that the body is retaining them unnaturally, inevitably producing harmful and toxic effects. Taking in what one needs is essential; getting rid of what one does not need is essential also.

BREATHING

We should pay special attention to our breathing. Proper inhalation is as important to health as taking in good food. The vital *Ch'i* energy is replenished not only by the food we eat, from our 'mother' earth, but also by the air that we breathe, from our 'heavenly father'. Time spent each day being conscious of our breathing, of taking in fresh air, is well spent. Also exhalation, another aspect of elimination. We need to breathe out properly; ridding ourselves of wastes, toxins and tensions will help us enormously.

EXERCISE

We should give due consideration to exercise, and finding our own ways of taking it. Walking is perhaps the best way of all but there are many other enjoyable ways – various sports, or dancing, or *tai chi*. In China, almost the whole population, young and old, can be seen in the early morning, out on the streets and in the squares and parks doing *tai chi* exercises. Exercise helps to improve circulation, breathing and elimination; above all, it helps quieten and calm the mind and emotions.

MODERATION IN OUR HABITS

We must not become slaves to our habits. The occasional cigarette or cigar, or the occasional alcoholic drink at a social gathering, these will do us no harm at all. After a demanding day, some people find that a smoke or a drink helps them to relax, a means of releasing tension. But moderation is the key.

All too often, if we don't keep a strict watch on ourselves, we find moderation giving way to excess. We begin to subject our bodies to more stress, rather than relieving it of tension. This tendency towards excess applies to many things – too many late nights, too many parties, too much entertaining and entertainment, too much television, too much physical work or exercise, too much mental work, too much talking, too much eating, too much sleeping. All such excesses can lead to ill health.

So our aim should be moderation – neither to forbid ourselves pleasures completely nor to indulge in them excessively. Obviously there will be certain situations where something has to be forbidden, usually where a severe state of imbalance has already been reached. With care, such situations will not develop.

THE FINDING OF AN INDIVIDUAL BALANCE

Each of us is different from everyone else. What may be right for one person can be wrong for another. Each must try to discover the needs of his or her own body, mind and spirit, and use common sense to keep within recognized limitations. It is not necessary to become fanatical and go through life worrying about whether one should or should not do this or that. The body is a remarkably resilient organism and is able to cope with most occasional stress and strain.

Further, I would add that I have found in my experience that outlook plays an important part in the finding of inner balance. If people begin to pay a little less attention to their own concerns and concentrate that bit more on helping others, they in turn grow a little stronger and healthier. Finding balance in that respect strengthens spirit and mind, and this in time is reflected in the body's health.

THE EDUCATION OF OUR CHILDREN

We can, if we wish, take the time and trouble to teach our children, from a very early age, the importance of moderation and of striving for a healthy body, mind and spirit. To over-indulge a child in any way in his formative years is to lead him into habits which can only be injurious to his health. Children should learn about the wonders of the mechanism of the body, and its closely-linked relationship with the mind, the environment and the whole creation. They should learn that the great riches of life are those that are freely given to us all, and that the opportunity is theirs to enjoy all such God-given blessings.

If they are brought up to follow 'the right way' – to try to live in harmony with the natural cycles and rhythms, to pay attention to the messages from their own minds and bodies, to observe and consider the effects on their health of their life style and their environment, and to respond and act according-ly – their lives should be long, rich and happy. They have the potential for being happy and healthy in almost any situation – if they gain a true sense of values, understand that happiness is not dependent on position, wealth and material things, and realize that the quality of life cannot be measured in years, only in the richness of each moment.

HEALTH CARE IN THE MODERN WORLD

If we are endeavouring to take care of ourselves and yet we still have various symptoms of trouble, albeit only minor, then it is best to get advice and treatment. A problem diagnosed and treated early means that less damage will have been done and that it will be much easier to correct.

This is where traditional Chinese acupuncture comes into its own and why it is one of the most beautiful methods of healing in the world. Its methods of diagnosis and treatment are available to help people to move back towards health before disease seriously develops.

It must be made quite clear, however, that acupuncture alone cannot prevent disease. The practitioner can diagnose disease developing and can help to trace causative and precipitating factors in the person's lifestyle. He can then give treatment to the person to help fight the disease. But, for improvement to be maintained, the causative factors in the person's life must be rectified by the person himself or herself.

The technological age, for all its advances, has created its own considerable threats and hazards where health and well-being are concerned. It is only by understanding the problems, and by people uniting in attempts to resolve them, that we shall be able to restore better conditions for better health.

As I have said, the Chinese saw man as a part of everything, of the whole creation, and as affected by everything in creation. They had great respect for Nature and its changing conditions, and hence placed emphasis on living by natural laws.

The state of their environment is of vital importance when considering the health of people. The acupuncture practitioner cannot treat them as if they live, as it were, in a vacuum. They have to be made well and kept well in relationship with their environment – within their own society and way of life. In order to lessen the causative factors of illness, it has to be part of the practitioner's duty to point out when necessary where people's way of living is causing ill health and to urge them to take action to rectify the situation.

Much has already been written about problems of environment and the Western way of life. The subjects are so crucial to health, however, that I feel they should be mentioned briefly. For example, we should ask ourselves how we are affected by 'high' standards of living, by growing world-population, by the arms and space race, and so on, purely from the standpoint of their effects on our health.

In the last decade or so, there has been a growing appreciation of ecological dangers; and some things have been done to deal with threats to health. Nevertheless, much more needs to be done on a larger scale. We all have responsibility not only for our own health but also for the health of everyone living in the world today. Our actions now have wider effects on the rest of the world than ever before. Activities in space, nuclear armament, scientific research – all can affect the whole planet. Disposal of toxic wastes becomes a matter of concern for everybody. The question is, do we have the right to advance our industry and manufacture if the resultant wastes pollute the atmosphere and the oceans of the world, endangering the health of present and future generations?

It is essential that each and every one of us should be concerned for the present and future health of the world. It is not enough for just the people working in medicine and related professions to be concerned about health hazards. All of us need to work together – including the politicians, industrialists, scientists, researchers – and to take a very careful look at the possible consequences of our actions in this modern day and age.

There is no question that our environment is no longer a healthy one; or, at least, that it is not as healthy as it was. Neither, in general, is our way of life a healthy one; at least not as healthy as it used to be. There is too much unrest and turmoil all over the world, and anxiety because the threat of nuclear war hangs over us.

The medical world struggles to keep people well. Great advances are made in the field of medicine; and yet such advance is continually counteracted by the fact that the Western way of life is driving people towards illness.

A vital part of the acupuncturist's work is to keep pointing to these causes of disease and asking patients to take note. Western attitudes will have to change considerably if we are to prevent escalation of disease. Society as a whole must be made much more aware of the effect on health of our way of living with all its attendant stresses. Society will have to be willing to make, and pay for, certain changes in modern lifestyle. If this becomes a priority, then improvements can be made.

To sum up, therefore, on health care in the modern world, there are three principal ways in which acupuncture can make a positive contribution:

(1) by traditional diagnosis – which can detect the cause of any imbalance in the energy of organs and functions, thus foreseeing disease before it manifests in the body, mind and spirit;

(2) by treatment – which aims to correct this imbalance by treating its cause before it has time to develop as disease;

(3) by teaching – which gives guidelines to living in ways which will encourage improved health. I hope it will be evident that the ancient Chinese teachings in this respect are as applicable today as they ever were.

Do you see this teaching about healthy living as part of the work of the acupuncturist today? Is not his time fully occupied in trying to restore the sick to health?

This is certainly a problem for the present–day practitioner. Very often, much as he would like to spend time helping and guiding people who are at present well but are seeking advice, in the main he is bound to feel that the seriously sick person who has turned to him for help must take priority. In general, it is only in small ways, at present, that acupuncture is able to carry out its teaching role for the improvement of general health.

The aim to act as counsellor and teacher – thus to improve health generally – was always a very important one for the true practitioner of traditional Chinese acupuncture. The scope of medical science in ancient China was very broad. This can perhaps be demonstrated by mentioning briefly a passage in the *Nei Ching,* the book that remains the foundation of traditional Chinese acpuncture. The Yellow Emperor, talking to his First Minister, Ch'i Po, sought instruction on all questions of health and the art of healing. He urged Ch'i Po to tell him about Nature, Heaven and the *Tao* (the Way), and asked to be informed about their workings. He wished to understand the workings to the utmost degree, including full information about man, his physical form, his blood, his breath of life, his flowering and his dissolution. He wanted to know what caused his death and his life, and he wished for advice on what should be done about all these things. Such was the range of knowledge expected in medical teaching.

This example gives just a glimpse of the Chinese concept of medicine. It could not in those days be studied as a particular and separate physical science. It was a science embracing Man's understanding of life and of all creaton. The art of healing involved philosophy and religion, both of which advocated oneness with Nature and the universe. Thus, the man of medicine had to study and understand the ancient philosophy which contained the three basic ideas inherent in all Chinese culture – the *Tao, Yin* and *Yang,* and the Five Elements. He had to concern himself with all such knowledge, as well as with anatomy and physiology, if he was to gain the necessary wisdom and understanding to heal body, mind and spirit.

The master of acupuncture was therefore much more than simply a medical man. He concerned himself with welfare in all respects. He was guide, mentor and instructor, helping people to follow a way of life which would keep their bodies, minds and spirits at all times in close harmony with natural law, and with the whole creation.

Even today, despite the absence of such concepts in the modern world, the traditional acupuncturist should keep them in mind and bring them to bear in the treating of patients.

12   The Training and Qualifications of a Practitioner

How long must one train to become proficient in the art of traditional Chinese acupuncture?

Traditional Chinese diagnosis can in fact 'take a lifetime' to master fully. By this I mean it can take that long to develop completely all the diagnostic skills – for example, to be able to read the twenty-eight different qualities of each of the twelve pulses, to see the facial colours clearly, and to distinguish sounds of the voice, odours, and emotions deeply and precisely. It takes a long time also to achieve facility with the whole range of acupuncture's therapeutic techniques. But, in practice, it is fair to say that a minimum of three years' training is necessary to achieve sufficient competence to practise. There are, as in other systems of medicine, several definite grades of proficiency.

At the College of Traditional Chinese Acupuncture, we grant a Licentiate certificate after a training period of three years. Any person receiving this certificate (Lic.Ac.) has been judged competent to give acupuncture treatment. The Licentiate will have undergone first, second and third year theoretical and practical examinations, and will have done one year's clinical training under supervision.

The majority of Licentiates then choose to continue their studies. The Lic.Ac. degree being the basic minimum requirement, they are encouraged to study the art in greater depth, and such is the fascination of this system of medicine, most of them are keen to continue. Each subsequent qualification (B.Ac., M.Ac., etcetera) is proof of the practitioner's continued study, experience and understanding.

Training for this system of medicine is not based on intellectual ability alone, important as this is; more important is the ability to develop sensitivity to life and to understand the philosophy which underlies traditional Chinese medicine. It really is true that a practitioner needs to continue to study for the rest of his life, such is the depth of the wisdom behind this system of medicine. He or she never stops learning.

So the majority of our Licentiates go on to try to attain a Bachelor degree. This takes a further two years of training, the main emphasis being on clinical diagnosis and practice. Successful candidates for this degree may then be invited to continue for a further two years in order to attain a Master's degree. As with training for the Bachelor degree, this course is primarily clinically orientated. Examinations during both of these degree courses are held at the end of the first and second years, and degrees are only awarded on successful completion of clinical training and examination. Finally, practitioners are then permitted to apply to take the Doctoral course, which lasts for three years. This is the final degree awarded by the College, and it indicates a minimum of ten years' training since the date of enrolment at the College.

In chapter 10, I explained at some length about the limitations of symptomatic acupuncture and about the dangers of acupuncture being practised by people without adequate knowledge of the tradition. I can only repeat that it is not safe to receive treatment from such inadequately trained people. Acupuncture treatment is capable of doing great good; but, if wrongly applied, it can also do harm.

It should therefore be borne in mind, when seeking a practitioner, that some people giving acupuncture treatment (including many orthodox doctors in their practices and in hospitals) have only received very short training and only have very limited knowledge and understanding of acupuncture. These people are usually unaware that they have had totally inadequate training and are usually ignorant of the dangers of practising it in that situation. A number of the students who pass through our College are Western doctors, and they need the same number of years training as all other students.

How does one know if the practitioner offering treatment is properly qualified?

The two things that you look for in choosing a practitioner are, first, that he or she is traditionally trained and has appropriate certificates of qualification, and, second, that he or she is well-recommended by people you trust. Like choosing any other professional adviser – a solicitor, a dentist, an accountant, or a vet – it is also a case of finding someone you get on with and feel you can trust.

No matter what the qualifications are, you can also consider the following guidelines, which act as an added safeguard and assurance that a practitioner is competent, thorough and careful.

How long did the practitioner take for the initial examination? If it was less than an hour you might have cause to be doubtful as to the quality of subsequent treatment. Did the practitioner read the pulses frequently? A good acupuncturist needs to read the pulses at least before and after every treatment. You might also ask yourself whether the practitioner concerned himself with all aspects of your welfare and health (and did not merely direct attention and treatment to the main symptom).

In this country there are at present three colleges whose training programmes in traditional Chinese acupuncture seek to match the standards of Chinese teaching hospitals.

Obviously, I can best speak for my own College which was established at Royal Leamington Spa in the early 1960's. It was the first college of traditional Chinese acupuncture opened specifically for training Westerners in strictly traditional methods. Since then, many students have passed the College's examinations and are now registered practitioners. The majority are practising in England; others are in practice in various countries worldwide.

The other two colleges are the International College of Oriental Medicine and the British Acupuncture Association.

Their graduates are also trained traditionally to a professional standard and have degrees similar to those mentioned above.

As a further safeguard of standards in the United Kingdom, there is a society of professional acupuncturists called the Traditional Acupuncture Society. Any graduate of The College of Traditional Chinese Acupuncture holding a Licentiate or higher qualification is eligible for nomination as a member (M.T.Ac.S.) or an associate member (A.T.Ac.S.).

The Society seeks to maintain standards appropriate to a responsible health care profession and its members are bound by a strict professional code of ethics. This code is a safeguard for the public and ensures the integrity of the Society's members. It is possible to obtain the names of registered practitioners, and the area where they work, by writing to the Secretary, Traditional Acupuncture Society, 11 Grange Park, Stratford-upon-Avon, Warwickshire.

The British Acupuncture Association and the International College of Oriental Medicine also have professional societies and registers of their qualified practitioners. The three organisations are at present working together, and are in the process of agreeing a common standard of education and professional care. They have jointly issued a Code of Practice for all practitioner members and have published a National Register of Acupuncturists (containing the names of all qualified practitioners of all three Societies) which may be obtained from any one of them.

It should be added, finally, that there are also in this country practitioners who have been trained abroad. Probably the only guidance and safeguard in these cases is to ascertain the extent of their training. Anything less than three years devoted to the study of acupuncture is most likely to have been inadequate and, of course, their methods of diagnosis and treatment should be in accord with traditional Chinese medicine. Qualifications in other fields of medicine do not make a person competent to practise acupuncture.

· Although acupuncture is an independent and separate medical science, it is recognised that practitioners in the West need to have a sound knowledge of orthodox anatomy, physiology and pathology. All three of the above-mentioned colleges either insist on new students having certificates of qualification in these subjects or the subjects are taught during the training course itself. As I mentioned earlier, all students of medicine in China now study these basic subjects before they proceed to specialize in either traditional Chinese medicine or in Western medicine.

13   Body, Mind and Spirit

In this final chapter, I would like to mention some of the deeper implications of what this little book is about. Brief references have been made to the *Tao* and to the importance of the spiritual aspects of life. I will try to bring these together to give better understanding of how man fits into the scheme of Nature.

Immediately I am faced with a difficulty – to talk about the *Tao* is to contradict its very existence. The Taoist sage Lao T'zu said that the *Tao* is The Way: it cannot be spoken about; it can only be lived.

Simply, the *Tao* may be seen as the way of being in accord with all of Nature in her fullest expression of harmony, beauty and wholeness. The Way that will bring fulfilment, happiness and health to body, mind and spirit depends on relating to the very essence of life in all its beauty. Traditional Chinese acupuncture helps cultivation of the *Tao*. It is a form of healing that is in tune with the *Tao;* its practice is ever-mindful and trusting that Nature, allowed to flow unimpeded, leads to health in body, mind and spirit, as Nature ordained it should be. It is resistance to and disobedience of the natural laws, the falling out of tune with Nature, that draws the lines on a man's brow, and withers his spirit. The *Tao* is more a way of the mind than the body, being the Way of realising the beauty and potential of the spirit within us all.

But what, then, is the spirit?

A lot of people feel uncomfortable when you mention the word 'spirit'. They think you are talking about some mystical entity, or are about to embark on some form of religious crusade. I feel personally that it is one of the great tragedies of the modern Western world that we have forgotten and ignore the real meaning and importance of the spirit. We claim to be at the peak of a civilizaton, but it is really a barbaric age we live in. Surely, if we were just a mind and a body, full stop, then we would be nothing more than clever robots? Technology has provided us with machines that are capable of 'thinking' and 'doing'; but what makes a human being a unique and wonderful individual? What gives that essential quality and spark to human life – its experience of ultimate joy, understanding and compassion? That *is* the spirit. But what importance do we attach to it today? I regret, hardly any at all.

We measure a child by its physical growth in its early days; 'Oh, hasn't the baby grown!' we say. Later, we measure by its mental development: 'Do you know, my son is now two books ahead of the rest of the class!'. This is how we take pride – boasting the development of physical body and mental ability. So what about the most important aspect of the child? How much do we encourage the state of the child's spirit?

This ignoring of the spirit is why we are not winning the fight against disease. We are abandoning and neglecting the deepest and most essential part of Man. And, if the spirit within us is denied, then we will not keep in harmony and balance. Thus we will be more susceptible to disease.

Some will call this spirit 'God', and quite rightly so, for 'God' is within each one of us. I do not mean some imaginary mythical or supernatural being, but your own 'God' within, call it what you wish. The ultimate. The creator of the whole universe. Not 'somebody' out there in the sky, or locked away in a church, but the divine spirit within each one.

Thus, in spite of all the so-called 'advances' made by science and technology, medical or otherwise, the incidence of disease is growing. It seems that today, more than at any time in the past, we are leading our lives in such a way that we are putting out our own fire, and all that that element represents. We are pushing into the background our natural and spontaneous expressions of love, joy, compassion, understanding and forgiveness. The greatest single thing that every human *needs* (and I distinguish intentionally here from 'desires'), more than anything else in the world, is *to be loved,* and *to love.* We cannot give priority to anything above that need because love is the very fuel of our lives and, if the Fire element becomes imbalanced, the fire starts to go out. The person loses the ability to love anyone, or to be loved by anyone, or to love himself or herself. Then there cannot be forgiveness, compassion or understanding. How many people today must be living totally barren lives because they have no loving exchange? Indeed, what is the point of going through life if you cannot love anybody, or if no one loves you? We have got to stop such foolish negligence of body, mind and spirit, and pay more attention to their needs, rather than striving excessively for status and wealth. Neither of these things in itself brings joy or fulfilment; but greed for them ends in sickness.

Certainly we realize the importance of giving love to a child; but then, when we are grown up, we seem to think our needs are so different. We can learn so much from the ancient wisdom of the Chinese who realised the truth in this matter. We all know how, when we are young, we depend upon our physical mother to love and feed us, and our physical father to guide and protect us. But when the day comes to leave our parents, we forget that we only stay alive thanks to our 'mother earth' and our 'father in the heavens', who, between them, provide the food that we eat (that which sustains us) and the air we breathe (that which inspires us), until the day that we die. So, like the Chinese, we should remember that all human beings are 'children' always, irrespective of age, and that we should take care to love and respect our Natural Parents, just as we did our physical parents, for without them we will surely perish.

Realizing these truly spiritual priorities gives us a nice and natural sense of proportion. We do not have to play adult games, pretending to be grown up, and striving to achieve grown-up aims. We can be happy in the way we were happy and content as children. A feeling of humility comes out of this understanding, so that we can begin to let go of our feelings of self-importance. The fact that all human beings have the same 'mother earth' and 'father in the heavens' means that we really are all brothers and sisters in the family of humanity – a family in which all are equal, and in which care should be given for one another.

Thus, the practitioner of traditional Chinese acupuncture does not claim his position to be special, nor does he claim the ability to cure. Rather, the practitioner is a servant of Nature, labouring on behalf of all her children, as a humble instrument assisting restoration of balance and harmony in body, mind and spirit.

Appendix One
Effects of the Western Way of Life on Health

I mentioned earlier in the book that our Western way of life places upon us great strains and pressures which lead to ill health and the lowering of resistance to disease. I left this statement largely unsupported because so much has already been written on the subject. However, as the state of our environment and our way of life play so vital a part in our general health, I feel it is important to append some further general observations.

I would say that there are three principal ways in which Western civilisation is presently exposing all of us to situations which can only be conducive to ill health.

First, we have a way of life in which we are persuaded to pursue an ever-higher standard of living. Our whole economy is geared to this escalation and all the power and resources of science and technology are applied to achieving this end. There is a general belief that more wealth will bring greater happiness. In our anxiety to provide all with ever-increasing material comforts, we have built up an environment which reveals a whole new generation of problems and pressures.

Second, there is the density of urban population, which affects people both physically and mentally. There are the direct effects on the body of convenience foods, re-cycled water and impure air, and all the mental pressures generated by the attempt to satisfy the needs and desires of large numbers of people and by their having to live in such close proximity to each other.

Third, there is the dominating influence of the international arms race, threatening our society with still further danger of destruction and pollution. Anxiety in this respect causes further mental stress.

THE PURSUIT OF HIGH STANDARDS OF LIVING

Of course, we all like the comforts and conveniences made possible by a high standard of living. People like holidays abroad, colour televisions, and the like. But we must take into account the detrimental effects of a spiralling and apparently insatiable demand for yet higher standards of living, and ask ourselves whether we can continue to afford it. This escalating demand for commodities must lead to bigger industry which in turn leads to more pollution, more stressful working conditions and depletion of resources. The insatiable pursuit also gives rise to all manner of tensions and conflicts within families and in personal relationships.

INDUSTRIAL POLLUTION

We pour our poisons and wastes from factories into rivers, lakes and seas. We discharge them into the air, and bury them beneath the earth. We seal toxic waste into containers and dump it out of sight. In transporting the raw materials and products, we foul the air with exhaust fumes and the sea with oil and sludge. There is virtually nowhere on this earth that remains unpolluted. The ecologists call constantly for immediate action but the steady poisoning of our environment continues, spelling distress and death to one form of life after another.

Until recently, it has been maintained that we cannot afford to deal satisfactorily with these dangerous side-effects of industry because it would be too expensive. Somehow we have also managed to persuade ourselves that, though other creatures and plants may be affected, Man will escape unscathed.

In the present trend of mass production and high consumption, it becomes too expensive to repair or re-use articles, and more and more are wastefully thrown away. Thus, the demand for raw materials increases – so that depletion of resources becomes even more serious – and the disposal of masses of rubbish results in more pollution.

Unemployment, with all of the emotional and mental strain that accompanies it, is an increasing problem. People begin to feel fortunate to have a job at all; but the satisfaction of having a job does not eliminate the problem of job satisfaction. Few workers in industry can be said to enjoy their work. Monotony is one considerable difficulty, and the shift system, in which workers are expected to be able to work, eat and sleep at any time of the day or night, is another.

This working situation places both physical and mental stress and strain on people. As a result, we have political conflict and industrial unrest – strikes, slowdowns, demands for more pay, for shorter hours, for more holidays, and so on. When people are subjected to such pressures year after year, they understandably get depressed and run down, and then turn to props or escapes of one sort or another. They drink too much, smoke too much, and take drugs or pills of every description – stimulants, tranquilizers, sleeping pills, vitamin pills, indigestion pills and headache pills.

People who are not getting satisfaction from their work, or do not have work, have to look for enjoyment elsewhere. The result is excessive entertainment and pleasure-seeking – with its consequent tendency to lowering of moral standards, to the debasing of sex, to adopting irresponsible attitudes to law and order and to a propensity for mindless and vicious violence. Anarchy comes uncomfortably closer.

EFFECTS ON THE INDIVIDUAL

Society's unrelenting drive for a higher standard of living seriously affects the individual. All too often the whole of a person's daily life is taken up with the pursuit and acquisition of wealth and material things. He or she is tempted by a hundred and one attractively-presented, skilfully-advertised articles and commodities. Desire to acquire them for self and family drives people along, often making them unrealistically ambitious, and leaving them no time to realise that they are caught up in the rat-race.

The common man rises from his bed, dashes to work, races

home at night, eats a meal in front of the television, goes to bed, only to repeat the same performance the next day. He lavishes time and affection on his car, his home, his furniture and his other possessions, often at the expense of his health. He is apparently prepared to sacrifice and abuse himself continually in order to achieve endless material gain.

PRODUCTION OF FOOD

The continuous and increasing demand for food has far-reaching detrimental effects. The primary object of agricultural production becomes quantity not quality, and questionable methods are used to obtain the highest possible yield of crops and livestock. The land is saturated with chemical fertilisers. The run-off of chemicals into waterways causes toxicity, and slowly life in the water is killed. Rivers and lakes become 'dead', devoid of life. Vegetables, fruit and cereal grains are sprayed against pests and disease; many of the chemicals used are poisonous. Much of our meat and poultry comes from 'factory' farms where the animals are confined in intensive-feeding units and never live in natural conditions. They are fed on artificially-boosted foods, and on antibiotics and other drugs which prevent the diseases they become susceptible to under such conditions. These antibiotics and drugs pass into the meat, milk, butter, cheese and eggs that we eat.

There is also continuous and increasing demand for water. It is needed in such large quantities that much of it has to be taken from polluted rivers. It then has to be purified with such chemicals as chlorine. Fluoride is also added because we insist on feeding ourselves and our children with foods guaranteed to cause tooth decay.

In order to feed urban concentrations of people there is also continuous and increasing demand for convenience foods – pre-prepared, processed, reconstituted, pre-cooked, etcetera. As do many of the less-obviously-processed foods, convenience foods contain all kinds of additives – artificial flavourings, colourings, sweeteners, laboratory-made vitamins, preservatives, and so on. Many of these have now been shown to be carcinogenic (cancer forming) after prolonged intake.

Obviously, our bodies depend on the food we eat and the air we breathe to provide vital fuel. Food and air supply our energy, the *Ch'i* energy. But practically all the food we eat today contains some unnatural substance, and no air anywhere in the world is entirely unpolluted. Thus our bodies are subjected to extra strain. Some of the unnatural substances taken in may be toxic, some may not; but all have to be coped with by our bodies.

AIR POLLUTION

Among the most serious causes of air pollution are the exhaust fumes of cars and other vehicles. And, of course, as the population's wealth increases, so does the number of vehicles.

Lead is one of the most dangerous constituents of exhaust fumes. Even at the North Pole, the lead content of the air is significant. And research in Europe has shown that lead, along with carbon monoxide, is having an insidiously harmful effect on city-dwellers, causing general malaise, headaches, depression and fatigue. The carbon monoxide is harmful to all life. Already, in certain areas of California, defoliation – due to high levels of this gas – is spreading rapidly.

It would be relatively easy to eliminate the lead problem. Removal of the carbon monoxide is more difficult. One method which has been found cuts down the quantity of carbon monoxide produced but increases the amount of nitrogen oxide. This gas is no less objectionable in that, in time, it affects the quality of sunlight reaching the surface of the earth. Unfortunately, cars using this method are actually in production. If we continue to pollute the atmosphere at the present rate, we will gradually build up our own fatal screen of death!

WASTES

Ever-increasing amounts of sewage and detergent have to be dealt with; much still goes straight into rivers and seas. Increasing amounts of household rubbish create disposal problems in towns and cities, especially the large quantities of waste plastic which, if burned, gives off toxic gases.

LOSS OF COUNTRYSIDE AND GROWING URBANISATION

More and more of the countryside is taken for town and road development and for vast reservoirs. Increasng numbers of people find themselves living in sprawling urban development, being further and further cut off from open country, fresh air and space. Studies of animal behaviour show that pressure of numbers in confined space creates such stress that it leads to irritability and fighting. Normal behaviour patterns become completely upset. There is no reason to suppose that man should respond any differently when living in confined space in close proximity to thousands of others.

NOISE

Noise is an ever-increasing and invasive stress factor. Thousands of people are subjected daily to severe stress through living and working close to streets, highways and airports. The modern way of life demands mobility, and the resulting aircraft and traffic noise creates a serious health hazard. The continuous noise of towns and cities disturbs the environment in which more and more people have to live.

HAZARDS OF THE ARMS RACE

During the period of frequent nuclear testing, alarming effects were noted: levels of radioactivity in the atmosphere were rapidly becoming dangerous to life on earth, radioactive fallout was found thousands of miles from the test sites and considerable atmospheric disturbances were recorded. High levels of surface radioactivity even occurred after underground tests. As a result of those nuclear tests, people now run a higher risk of bone cancer, leukemia and thyroid trouble than previous generations.

Meanwhile, enormous stockpiles of various weapons periodically become obsolete and have to be 'disposed of' somewhere. It is chilling to remember, for example, the proposal by the United States Government to dump 27,000 tons of nerve gas in the Atlantic Ocean – a proposal which, thankfully, caused raging controversy.

An over-riding cause of anxiety and stress, however, arises from the fact that there is always the danger of something going wrong in research with modern methods of warfare, nuclear or otherwise. In Skull Valley, Utah, six thousand sheep were accidentally killed as a result of United States Army tests of the nerve gas 'Vx'. The dangerous effects of biological or chemical warfare are said to exceed even those of nuclear warfare. It was reported in *The Times* (4th July 1969) that Guinard, an island off the north-west coast of Scotland, was experimentally infected with anthrax. This proved so successful that it would be fatal for up to the next hundred years for anyone to live there. On another occasion, scientists from all over the world warned the United States of the possibly-irreparable damage that might be done through putting vast quantities of experimental 'needles' into space, for some military defence project. The American military advisers chose to ignore these warnings and urged approval of the scheme. The 'needles' went up (with as yet unknown consequences).

It is shortsighted and foolish in the extreme that the fears one nation has of another should prompt it to act in such a way as to endanger the balance (and existence) of life on this earth, and the balance of the earth in relaton to the cosmos. Very little is known of the possible consequences on the biosphere and stratosphere of many of our arms race (and space) experiments. Whatever these consequences may be, the majority of us have to live with the anxiety that they could be catastrophic.

EFFECTS ON MENTAL HEALTH

Apart from its insidious effect on adults, the arms race has had and is having a hard-to-measure yet real effect on the mentality of young people. Overwhelmed by the apparent pointlessness of living, due to the threat of mass destruction, many young people have suffered, and continue to suffer, a depression and lethargy born of fear. Others have become belligerent and anarchistic in their frantic determination to break down the structures and attitudes of a society which seems to condone the arms race and to ignore the possible consequences.

Most important and dangerous of all – in this fear, confusion and mad chase after material comfort – is the fact that Man's spiritual needs may be overlooked or pushed into the background. Modern scientific and technological knowledge tends to persuade us that there is no need for religion, that it is all myth and superstition. We are encouraged instead to put our trust in secular 'isms' – materialism, behaviourism, humanism, realism, atheism, pragmatism, agnosticism, existentialism and the like. It is my own personal opinion – but I'm sure I am not alone in this – that Man's sickness will continue to increase until he stops seeking happiness in possessions and transient pleasures, and stops seeking to defend them at any cost.

Each and every one of us, sometime during our lives, experiences that deep peace and love, joy and fulfilment, which comes from within. We should cease looking for them outside ourselves, and acknowledge gratefully that they arise from the 'Kingdom of God' within.

But, herewith, more than ever, I need to emphasize the truth that a healthy body, mind and spirit depend on moderation. Far be it from me to suggest that science and technical advancement should be totally discarded, any more than I would suggest that the spiritual needs of man and woman should be exclusive of earthly needs. The need is for moderation in both, for an acknowledgement, reconciliation and respect of both; but *never* for one to be to the detriment or exclusion of the other.

Appendix Two
Acupuncture in the United States of America

Traditional Chinese acupuncture is not just a skill or a science that can be learnt solely from books. As you will have seen throughout this book, it is a way of Nature, a way of understanding the energies that govern body, mind and spirit.

Traditionally, knowledge was passed verbally from father to son. The lessons were taken from Nature, not from books. The skill and expertise came from observation and experience. In this twentieth century we have to try our best, whilst maintaining all that is precious within traditional Chinese acupuncture, to impart this knowledge through schools and colleges. Much good work can be done in this way, not least through being able to share understanding of the basic laws and rules, and all the complex and subtle aspects with which a student of acupuncture needs to be familiar.

Because I believe and know the teachings of *traditional* Chinese acupuncture to be true, I am apprehensive in that this classical system faces a dilemma in this day and age. Modern sociological, educational and political forces threaten its survival. It is in danger of becoming distorted through some peoples' endeavours to make it fit modern scientific structures, methods, and systems.

Understanding and practice of traditional acupuncture in Europe is many generations ahead of the United States of America, and is is in the United States of America that these political and educational forces are more seriously undermining the classical tradition.

During a lecture tour in the United States in the early part of 1970, I toured many universities and hospitals and made a considerable number of radio broadcasts and appearances in television programmes throughout the country. Acupuncture was then a new word representing, to the vast majority of people, a strange and foreign method of healing.

There were, at that time, some Chinese people in their own communities who were practising forms of acupuncture; but, excluding them, only one or two Americans in the whole of the States were practising. Then came the visit of President Nixon to China, and, on his return, a floodgate of publicity seemed to open, extolling the virtues of Chinese medicine. Within a very short time, there were numerous organizations offering one-day courses, two-day courses, one-hundred-hour courses, certifying people on completion as proficient in the art. The people who were running these courses had next to no knowledge about traditional practice. Fortunately, the situation has now passed and such practices made illegal.

Those well-trained practitioners who felt there was a rightful place for this system of medicine to be taught and practised properly in America then had to turn their energies to getting laws altered and passed which would enable them to practise good acupuncture legally. It is a great credit to these people that they were able to muster the energy to lobby successfully the necessary Congressmen and Senators to give them recognition. Legal status has now been achieved in certain States. Personally I regard with admiration these persevering efforts.

However, this process has given rise to the dilemma I mentioned at the beginning. In order to obtain the necessary legal status, many compromises have had to be made to meet sociological, educational and political requirements. There has been some detraction from the essence and principles of the system as it should be practised. It is here that I am fearful – that much more still may have to be sacrificed in order to fit the traditional system into the modern, technological age.

That being said, standards are improving each year, and now, some ten years after President Nixon's visit to China, many States have proper examination procedures, ensuring that only qualified applicants are permitted to practise. Schools and colleges have been set up which endeavour to meet the minimum requirements laid down by State legislature.

However, as I say, some of these requirements are not ones which promote and encourage a standard of excellence in the *practise of traditional Chinese* acupuncture. The emphasis in these colleges, unfortunately, tends to be on theory and academic standards, and is very much directed towards passing the written State examinations. This is not a system of medicine that can be entirely taught in this way. But I have no hesitation in suggesting that in some fifteen years from now, it is possible that America will be the foremost country in the whole of the Western world in having acupuncture practice on an established footing.

What would break my heart would be to see this development threatened as a result of teaching by people who have little or no *practical* experience. The danger is that the teaching will lack the traditional essence, subtlety and spirit. It is too early to tell for sure if this will happen. One saving grace, I feel, is the tremendous respect so many American people have for natural laws. One can only hope that through their turning back to Nature, and rejecting man-made pollution, they will appreciate this natural system of medicine. They will then ensure that the people who are practising acupuncture are doing so with care and intelligence, and are properly qualified.

How does one find a traditionally-trained practitioner?

There are numerous practitioners (and teachers) in the United States of America who have been studying at the College in England for varying periods (from five to ten years). They are teaching acupuncture in a manner that preserves the traditional. Many of them are doctors who have had to undergo exactly the same training as the non-medical practitioner.

The addresses of all UK-trained graduates working in the States may be obtained by writing to the Registrar, The College of Traditional Chinese Acupuncture, Tao House, Queensway, Royal Leamington Spa, England; or to the Registrar and Secretary to the Council, The Traditional Acupuncture Society, 11 Grange Park, Stratford-upon-Avon, Warwickshire, England; or to the Registrar of the Traditional Acupuncture Institute, Room 108, American City Building, Columbia, Maryland.

This, of course, does not mean that there are no other practitioners in the United States of America who have undergone traditional training in other countries who are also competent to practise. But I can only speak for the ones whom I know about personally; beyond this recommendation it is up to those interested to investigate and evaluate for themselves, hopefully sufficiently informed as to what to look for by the content of this book.

An organization has also been formed called the National Council for Acupuncture Schools and Colleges (N.C.A.S.C.), and I understand it is this Council's intention to set up and preserve standards of competence and teaching through the whole of the United States of America to bring high standards and common purpose. It will be able to recommend the various teaching establishments and qualified practitioners as ones that conform to the Council's standards.

These establishments will, of course, incorporate the various educational, political and social requirements of each State but they will also safeguard the teachings, and thus the quality, of acupuncture in the United States. I wish this body every success as it offers a safeguard to the American public, and to sick people in particular.